SEATED ACUPRESSURE MASSAGE

From Ancient Art to Modern Practice

a practical guide for therapists

SEATED ACUPRESSURE MASSAGE

From Ancient Art to Modern Practice
a practical guide for therapists

**Patricia Abercromby and
Davina Thomson**

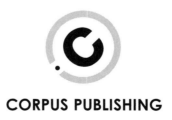

CORPUS PUBLISHING

First published in 2001 by
Corpus Publishing Limited
9 Roman Way, Fishbourne, Chichester, PO19 3QN

Author's note
As seated acupressure massage has its roots in both China and Japan, we have recognized this by using both Chinese and Japanese symbols in the first two chapters.

Disclaimer
This publication is intended as an informational guide. The techniques described are a supplement, and not a substitute for professional tuition. Whilst the information herein is supplied in good faith, no responsibility is taken by either the publisher or the author for any damage, injury or loss, however caused, which may arise from the use of the information provided.

British Library Cataloguing in Publication Data
A CIP record for this book is available from the British Library
ISBN 1 903333 01 6

Acknowledgements
I am grateful to all my clients of seated acupressure massage, who over the years have given me such satisfaction and made every day a new experience, often leaving me in awe with the profound and sometimes astounding results they have achieved from this therapy. I would also like to thank Patricia for her constant motivation and for always aiming for the summit.

Davina Thomson

We are both grateful to our families and friends who supported our efforts in putting this book together. I have benefited enormously from working with Davina whose experience in the classroom as a tutor, and as a working practitioner of seated acupressure massage are arguably, unsurpassed in this branch of complementary therapy.

Patricia Abercromby

Also, we are grateful to Mel Cash, Leon Chaitow, Maria Mercati, Shogo Mochizuki, Meir Schneider and Anne Silk for aspects of their wisdom and works that have contributed to this book, and in addition, to Anne Silk and Polly Harper for their guidance, encouragement and contributions.

Photography Keith Spillett
Drawings Dominic Harris
Text and Cover Design Bookman
Printed and bound in Great Britain by Bell & Bain Ltd., Glasgow
Distributed throughout the world by Human Kinetics - www.humankinetics.com - or:
USA
P O Box 5076, Champaign, IL 61825-5076 T: 1-800-747-4457 F: 217-351-1549
Canada
475 Devonshire Road, Unit 100, Windsor, ON N8Y 2L5 T: 1-800-465-7301 F: 519-971-9797
Australia
P O Box 80, Torrens Park, S. Australia 5062 T: (08) 8277-1555 F: (08) 8277-1566
UK and Europe
Units C2-C3 Wira Business Park, West Park Ring Road, Leeds, LS16 6EB, UK
T: +44 (0) 113 278 1708 F: +44 (0) 113 278 1709
New Zealand
P O Box 105-231, Auckland Central T: (09) 523-3462 F: (09) 523-5462

Contents

Foreword

Some books are written to fulfil the authors dreams or ambitions whilst others are the result of a genuine need to tell the story or impart vital information. We believe Seated Acupressure Massage by Patricia Abercromby and Davina Thomson falls magnificently into both categories.

We have known Davina Thomson and Patricia Abercromby for several years and have visited their successful school on a number of occasions. They are both passionate about 'their therapy' and nothing is too much trouble to ensure they produce well trained and competent practitioners. This passion and eye for detail shines through this book, which is well produced and a fine balance exists between graphical detail and precise instruction. One can actually 'see' their students working as you progress through the easy to read pages.

Davina has been teaching various aspects of massage for many years and is an experienced teacher. For the last few years she has concentrated in running courses in Seated Acupressure Massage ably assisted in both the administration and teaching by Patricia Abercromby, herself a qualified therapist and teacher.

The style of clothed and seated massage has gained popularity during the last ten years. The practitioner/therapist usually visits the workplace and many businesses find it beneficial for their employees, because it relaxes both mental and physical tensions thereby reducing stress and stress related problems and can create a measurable reduction in sick days.

This well written and illustrated book will be an excellent teaching aid to students and an aide-mémoire for the experienced practitioners. We found the chapters featuring the history of Acupressure Massage and the basic understanding of Traditional Chinese Medicine very interesting and the section devoted to helping the therapist promote and market their newly acquired skills in the world of business completes the reader's education. Destined to be a best seller in this specialist market.

Shirley and John Beney
The Guild of Complementary Practitioners

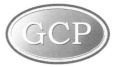

Introduction

Seated acupressure massage has entered into the culture not only as an acceptable modality in the corporate stress management environment, but also in the public sector. Go to any Health Fair or Exhibition and you will see seated acupressure massage practitioners working nonstop with a line of people waiting patiently for their 'turn.' In most major shopping malls, airports and fitness centres in many parts of the world, practitioners can be found demonstrating their skills on a willing and grateful public, and walk-in 'back rub' shops are opening up in many High Streets in cities and towns.

While it is a good development that so many people are willing to sit down on the ultra-comfortable massage chairs and receive a treatment, it is vitally important that members of the public can be confident that their practitioner is fully qualified and insured to practice. In the UK, there are only three training schools offering courses in seated acupressure massage that are fully accredited by the Guild of Complementary Practitioners. We would urge anyone who is considering training in this modality or any person seeking a treatment, to check the credentials of the training school and the qualifications of the practitioner offering the session.

We have included a detailed account of the 20-minute sequence that we teach in our school. There will be slight variations from sequences taught by other schools, but the basic KATA is instantly recognizable. Practitioners will find that working with clients sitting in the chair creates many possibilities for a variety of additional therapeutic and remedial techniques to enhance the basic sequence and to treat specific ailments, such as a range of overuse injuries. Some of our most frequently used additional techniques are included, but we are sure that you will have your own favourite and effective techniques to add to the list.

Marketing oneself as a practitioner is an area that traditionally, gives many of us some grief. We have tried to give practitioners a few hints and tips on how to sell themselves and their services to a potentially vast client base. Also included are ways for practitioners to look after themselves and ensure that they stay fit and healthy. After all, we need to practice what we preach!

Although no book or video can ever be a substitute for attending a structured training course, we hope that the contents of the following pages will build on the knowledge of qualified practitioners of seated acupressure massage and will inspire others to learn this exciting and dynamic skill.

Patricia Abercromby and Davina Thomson

Chapter 1
History of Acupressure Massage

The seated acupressure massage techniques that are taught and practised today have evolved from ancient East Asian massage techniques called ANMA in Japan, and ANMO in China. Anma translated literally, means press and rub, represented by the combination of Japanese characters for Anma.

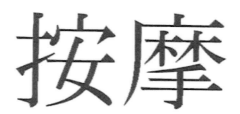

Japanese
Anma script

This tradition has survived thousands of years of being passed down through generations building on their observations of Yin and Yang concepts, the Five Element Theory, (more of that later) meridians and acupressure points. Ancient writings from Japan indicate that Anma has its roots in India, Nepal, Tibet and Western China dating back 7000 years.

There is an interesting legend that the Chinese came to understand the power of acupressure points with the arrival around 10000 BC, of incredible seven feet tall healers known as the Sons of Reflected Lights. These beings could see the aura and the meridians of people with the acupressure points showing up as tiny pinpricks of light. They healed by directing their own life force at the sick person from a distance of several feet. Over the centuries, their sensitivity and power decreased and they moved closer and closer to the body until they were using the pressure of their fingertips, eventually graduating to acupuncture needles. Perhaps difficult to prove without any documented evidence but it makes a nice story.

Anma massage was first recorded in China during the Zhou and Qin Dynasties (1122AD – 207AD). During the Han Dynasty (221BC – 264BC) the legendary visionary, the Yellow Emperor Huang Ti referred to Anma and Acupuncture in the Huang Ti Nei Ching or the Yellow Emperors Classic of Internal Medicine, now recognised as the oldest existing medical text in the world. Modern medical research has 'rediscovered' many of the medical observations made in this ancient tome and found them to be accurate. In the Huang Ti Nei Ching, it states that 'kidney supports bone', a truth somewhat lost on the Western medical establishment. This was until it was discovered that Vitamin D is an important factor in bone growth and more recently, that the chemistry of Vitamin D is changed in the kidney and provides the missing link in the control of bone growth and development.

Acupuncture became the treatment of choice for the Chinese nobility while the healers, or barefoot practitioners as they were known, travelled around from village to village offering Anma massage. Late in the Tang Dynasty which began in 618AD, the practice of Anma declined sharply but emerged later in Southern China as Tui-na, a form of Chinese massage that is growing in popularity in the West today.

In the early part of the fifth century, China started trading with Japan through Korea, and the Japanese were introduced to Buddhism and the art of Chinese medicine including Anma. In 718AD, a medical school was established in Japan to study acupuncture and Anma. More than 200 hundred years later, during which time many Chinese Buddhist monks and doctors emigrated to Japan, the oldest comprehensive medical text in Japan, the I Shin Bo was published in 984AD, covering all known medical subjects including Anma.

In spite of a decline in interest for a few hundred years between 1185 – 1574, the art of Anma survived and indeed flourished during the Monoyama period 1575 – 1602. Many new Anma techniques evolved during this time and were taught in the new medical schools that were established in Tokyo.

During the Edo period, 1602 – 1868 there was an exchange of medical knowledge with physicians who came to Japan with the Dutch Trading Company. The Dutch doctors introduced the Japanese practitioners to anatomy and physiology and in exchange, the Dutch doctors learned acupuncture and Anma and brought them back to Europe. Possibly as a result of this exposure to Western medicine, the powerful shoguns decreed in the middle of the 19th century, that only blind practitioners, who would have better developed touch sensitivity, should perform Anma for relaxation purposes. As the blind practitioners could not practise other forms of medicine such as herbalism, Anma massage came to be regarded as a poor person's health system and much technical and clinical knowledge was lost during this time.

Between 1868 – 1912, the shoguns fell from power to be replaced by an imperialistic government. Western medical practices became popular, to the detriment of traditional Oriental medicine. However, the blind Anma practitioners survived until the turn of the 20th century when the Japanese government of the day decreed that all Anma practitioners should be licensed and taxed. Many of them prudently reinvented themselves as Shiatsu (meaning finger pressure) practitioners to avoid the tax and licensing laws. In its early days a Shiatsu therapist performed only the Anma finger pressure but it has developed to include other areas of massage and Anma techniques. Shiatsu increased in popularity and was made more acceptable by Tamai Tempaku, a massage practitioner with a good knowledge of western anatomy and physiology and massage, who published a book in 1919 called Shiatsu Ho. In 1925, an Institute for Shiatsu was established by one of his students, Tokujiro Namikoshi. Massage was no longer restricted to the blind, and a more structured system of education and training was implemented for Anma and massage therapy. In 1964, Shiatsu was licensed as a therapy in its own right, independent from Anma.

Although Shiatsu evolved from Anma and both disciplines are similar in many respects, there are one or two differences to note. Anma utilises kneading and percussive movements not used in Shiatsu. Vibration techniques are used a lot in Anma but only occasionally in Shiatsu. Both techniques apply pressure to the acupressure points or tsubos, on the meridians.

Seated acupressure massage is a hybrid of both modalities and was developed specifically for the workplace, hence the popular name of 'on-site massage'. David Palmer, an American practitioner was the pioneer of seated acupressure massage in the West. In 1984 David was giving 15-minute massages through clothing to employees at Apple Computers in Silicon Valley in California. This was so well received that he went on to design a folding, portable massage chair. The chair provides total body support for the client and enables the practitioner to give a more therapeutic and effective treatment.

In 1989, the sequence was being taught in the UK and since then it has continued to grow in popularity in many countries throughout the world. In its present form, the basic sequence or KATA (Japanese for dance), takes 20 minutes to perform and works on many acupressure points on the upper body, including shoulders, upper and lower back, arms, hands, neck and head. Although there are some variations of the sequence as taught by different training schools, the basic sequence is instantly recognisable from the stance of the practitioner and from the meridians that are worked on. If a time machine could transport us back three thousand years to Japan or China, it is likely that the Anma practitioners of those times would recognise the modern seated acupressure massage sequence on offer today.

Chapter 2
An Overview of Traditional Chinese Medicine

Seated acupressure massage has its roots in ancient, traditional oriental massage techniques, and when practised with skill, accuracy and empathy, the 20-minute sequence will help balance the flow of energy or Qi throughout the body, as the practitioner stimulates many acupressure points on the 12 major meridians. This will happen without the practitioner necessarily having an in-depth knowledge of Yin and Yang and the Five Element Theory, the conceptual basis of Traditional Chinese Medicine, of which acupressure massage is an integral part. There are many excellent books available for those who wish to study this subject further. This chapter provides an introductory overview of the traditional Chinese view of health and disease, and hopefully, will give practitioners of seated acupressure massage, a better understanding of the multiplicity of factors, physical, emotional and environmental affecting their individual client's state of health.

The major difference between Chinese medicine and Western medicine is that Western medicine is based on a philosophy that views disease either as a physical or mental problem. Although there is a general assumption that the two may be loosely connected, Western medical doctors, in tandem with the pharmaceutical industry, normally treat symptoms individually.

Disease is approached from the view that it is caused by external factors such as invasion by bacteria or viruses or by degeneration of internal organs or systems of the body.

The philosophy of Chinese medicine is that everything in the Universe is part of an interdependent and mutually interactive energy force called Qi, where mind, body and spirit are merely different elements of the same life force and should not be considered separately.

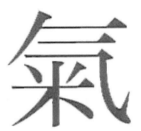

Universal Energy

Treatments seek to balance the energy dynamics, Yin and Yang, of the individual, by taking into consideration physical symptoms, emotional reactions and environmental factors. Thus a practitioner of Traditional Chinese Medicine (TCM), might use or suggest a combination of acupuncture, herbal remedies, Qigong exercises, meditation or a Feng Shui reading to bring balance and harmony to their patients' lives. The Chinese culture was one of the first to introduce preventative medicine where the wealthier patients visited their doctor when they were well, paying the doctor a retainer to keep them healthy. The doctor would lose his fee if his patient fell ill!

In spite of the radical differences between Chinese and Western medical systems, the two are not mutually exclusive, and elements of each can benefit the health of the individual. Practitioners of complementary therapies, including seated acupressure massage, are uniquely placed to bridge the gap between the two approaches and can help broaden the philosophical and ideological basis of Western and Chinese medicine.

Yin and Yang

The concept of Yin and Yang is about balance between opposites, and in the body, balance means good health. Yin represents water, quiet, substance and night while Yang represents fire, noise, function and day. In the body,

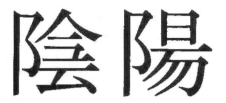 *Yin and Yang*

disease is caused by an imbalance of Yin and Yang. Therefore, disease can be treated by correcting this imbalance and allowing the body to heal itself. The Chinese physicians are great advocates of moderation in all things including alcohol and food.

Daily activities should include both physical and mental exercise. Each of the organs of the body has an element of Yin and Yang, although one will be more Yang than Ying. The meridians are paired in Yin and Yang, which is the representation of opposite but complementary qualities that are interdependent and are in a constant state of dynamic balance.

In a healthy body Qi circulates in a self-regulating balance. It is always moving, and there is a constant flow between two Yin and Yang meridian systems. They are opposite to each other but mutually dependent. For example, the lung meridian Yin and large intestine Yang, are paired, or sister meridians. Blocked energy in either meridian can create an imbalance in the associated organ systems.

If one sister meridian has an excess of energy, the other will have a deficiency, so stimulating one or both, can alleviate the imbalance. Sometimes the balance of Yin and Yang in a healthy body is not always exact. If a person is angry and fiery, that is Yang, but at other times, they may be quiet and reflective, that is Yin. If however, the person was permanently angry and fiery, there would be an excess of Yang and the body becomes unhealthy and disease results.

The Five Element Theory

The origins of Chinese philosophy, Taoism, developed through observation of the world. Everywhere in nature there is a dynamic interchange between Yin and Yang. The seed, Yin, grows into the plant, Yang, which in turn dies back into the earth, Yin. This growth takes place through the seasons, Winter, Yin, Spring and Summer, Yang and transforms through the

Autumn, back into Winter. Drawing on these observations in nature, the early Chinese Taoists developed a medical system known as the Five Element Theory. This gives a deeper explanation of how Qi balances, interacts and supports all life forms. The elements are the basis of all that exists: Metal, Water, Wood, Fire and Earth. Each element is part of a larger cycle of Universal energy that is constantly moving. The creation or Sheng cycle is the growth cycle and is placed in check by the control or Ke cycle. Unending growth would cause a compounding energy from one element to another and result in an extreme imbalance. The control cycle counteracts the creation cycle and restores balance and harmony. Each element corresponds to the natural world and to the human body, and this pattern of interrelationships is used as a model for the way in which the processes of the body support each other.

Arising from the Five Element Theory is the Cosmological Sequence with its origins in Chinese numerology. This places the Water Element at the root of the cycle. As the Water Element corresponds to the kidneys, they are considered in Chinese medicine to be the source of Yin/Yang energy in the body. The Spleen, at the centre of the Cosmological Sequence is considered to be the origin of Qi in the body and supports all the other organs.

Element	Paired or Sister Meridians	
	YIN	YANG
Metal	Lung	Large Intestine
Water	Kidney	Bladder
Wood	Liver	Gall Bladder
Fire	Heart	Small Intestine
	Heart Protector	Triple Heater
Earth	Spleen	Stomach

FUNCTIONS OF THE ORGAN SYSTEMS

Lung

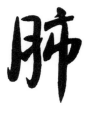

1. Regulates the secretion of sweat.
2 Regulates body hair and skin.
3. Respiratory conditions including asthma and coughing.
4. Eliminates noxious gases through exhalation.
5. Rules Qi and regulates Qi of entire body.

Large Intestine

1. Receives food and water from the small intestine and absorbs some of the fluids and excretes the remainder.
2. Removes stagnant Qi through excretion.
3. Supports lung in functions of respiration and immune system activities.
4. Elimination.

Kidney

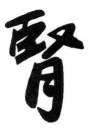

1. Governs 'Jing' essence, the substance that underlies all organic life (a reservoir that nourishes the body and fuels the metabolism – jing is primarily inherited but enhanced by nutrition, exercise and lifestyle).
2. Governs bones and marrow and teeth.
3. Proper functioning of the ears.
4. Memory and concentration.
5. Harmonising sexual functions.
6. Survival and instinctual fear.

Bladder

1. Transforms fluids through storage and excretion.
2. Helps to balance entire meridian system (through corresponding association points along meridian).
3. Addresses fear, depression, worry and agitation.

Gall Bladder

1. Regulates the flow of Qi throughout body.
2. Governs decision-making process.
3. Influences the eyes, ligaments, tendons and joints.
4. Excess gall bladder Qi, may be shown as anger and deficiency as timidity and depression.

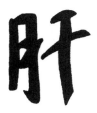

Liver

1. Maintains the harmonious movement of Qi throughout the body; known as the 'controller of strategic planning'.
2. The principal centre of metabolism – synthesising proteins, neutralising poisons, assisting in the regulation of blood sugar levels and secreting bile.
3. Harmonising emotions.

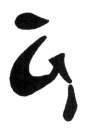

Heart

1. Governs the entire vascular system, controlling direction and strength of blood flow.
2. Nourishes tissues, removes toxins and influences all other organs.
3. Rules mental energy, known as Shen or Spirit.
4. Because of its importance it has a heart protector or pericardium.

Heart Protector (Pericardium)

1. Protects the heart from external stresses – on a physical and emotional level.
2. Supports the heart in circulatory functions.

Triple Heater

The triple heater is a function rather than an organ:

1. It transforms and transports Qi as it flows to all parts of the body and directs Qi to the organs, known as the 'Official of Balance and Harmony'.
2. Helps to transform and transport nourishment and to excrete waste.
3. Enhances the functions of the lymphatic system.

Small intestine

1. Responsible for receiving and transforming nourishment by absorbing food and drink.
2. Separating the pure or useful substances from waste products.
3. Assimilation of nutrients.
4. Rules discernment.

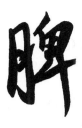

Spleen

1. Assists digestive process by transporting and transforming food.
2. Absorbing nourishment and sorting usable from unusable.
3. The primary organ in the production of prenatal Qi.
4. Ingested food and drink provide food Qi and creates postnatal Qi.
5. Governs blood, muscles, limbs and connective tissue – proper movement is dependent upon a well-balanced spleen meridian.

Stomach

1. Referred to as the 'sea of nourishment' in charge of digestion.
2. Transports food energy to all parts of body and nourishes muscles.
3. Whatever the disease, if stomach Qi is strong, the outlook is good.

The Governing Vessel is known as the 'sea of Yang channels', and influences all the Yang meridians and is used to enhance the body's Yang energy. It nourishes the brain and spine.

The Conception vessel is known as the 'sea of Yin channels'. It influences all the Yin meridians and is important for the reproductive system, fertility, pregnancy and conception.

Five Element Theory Summarised

CREATION (Sheng) CYCLE

Fire creates Earth	The ashes of fire add to earth
Earth creates Metal	The expansion of earth creates metal
Metal creates Water	Metal separates, allowing water to flow
Water creates Wood	Water nourishes the growth of wood
Wood creates Fire	Wood builds fire

CONTROLLING (Ke) CYCLE

Fire controls Metal	The heat of fire melts metal
Metal controls Wood	Metal can chop wood
Wood controls Earth	The roots of trees grow through earth
Earth controls Water	Earth can dam water
Water controls Fire	Water can dowse fire

Although wood controls earth it also builds fire which controls earth. This is a checks and balances system. In relation to acupressure, the Five Element Theory is the basis for determining how to re-balance energy and help the natural healing process. The five elements are assigned particular characteristics which provide information for the practitioner, i.e. colour, emotions, season, body parts, meridians, climate and seasons.

	YANG	**YIN**
In the world:	Sun	Moon
	Upper	Lower
	Hollow	Solid
	Positive	Negative
In the body:	Spine/back	Chest/abdomen
	Male	Female
	Surface of the body	Interior of the body
In dis-ease:	Acute	Chronic

Meridians and Acupressure Points

The meridians are a system of conduits that carry Qi or vital energy to every part of the body. There are twelve major meridians associated with an organ system with over 350 acupressure points and a further 250 non-meridian points. Disease is considered to be present when there is a disruption to the flow of energy through a channel. For instance, a sprain or strain injury will interrupt the flow of energy through the associated channel, or if there is an internal disruption of Yin and Yang balance and disease results, there will be an abnormal flow of energy through the channel associated with the diseased organ. As meridians cannot be identified in the same way as blood or lymph vessels, it is best to understand them as a process rather than as structures. The twelve major meridians are:

Lung Meridian	L
Large Intestine Meridian	LI
Stomach Meridian	ST
Spleen Meridian	SP
Heart Meridian	H

Small Intestine Meridian	SI
Bladder Meridian	BL
Kidney Meridian	KI
Triple Heater (Warmer) Meridian	TW
Heart Protector Meridian (Pericardium)	PC
Gall Bladder Meridian	GB
Liver Meridian	LV

The meridians form two symmetric loops on either side of the body and energy flows through them in a well-defined, 24-hour circadian rhythm. Two further meridians on the median line, the centre of the body, are the Conception Vessel meridian and the Governing Vessel meridian. The cycle flows from the chest area along the three inner arm (Yin) Lung, Heart Protector and Heart Meridians. Here they connect with the posterior arm (Yang) Large Intestine, Triple Heater and Small Intestine meridians and flow upwards to the head. From the head, they connect with leg (Yang) meridians, Stomach, Gall Bladder and Bladder and flow downwards to the feet. In the feet they connect with the leg (Yin) meridians, Spleen, Liver, Kidney and flow up to the chest to complete the cycle.

During the 24-hour cycle, there are specific times when there is a maximum flow of energy in each channel:

Lung Meridian	3 am – 5 am
Large Intestine	5 am – 7 am
Stomach Meridian	7 am – 9 am
Spleen Meridian	9 am – 11 am
Heart Meridian	11 am – 1 pm
Small Intestine Meridian	1 pm – 3 pm
Bladder Meridian	3 pm – 5 pm
Kidney Meridian	5 pm – 7 pm
Heart Protector Meridian	7 pm – 9 pm
Triple Heater Meridian	9 pm – 11 pm
Gall Bladder Meridian	11 pm – 1 am
Liver Meridian	1 am – 3 am

It is interesting to correlate this information with a recent French survey that showed accidents in the morning are more likely to happen if breakfast has been missed. A quick check with the above list shows that Qi is concentrated in the stomach meridian between 7 am and 9 am, so – don't skip breakfast!

Acupressure Points or Tsubos

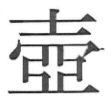 Tsubo, often translated as 'jar' or 'vessel,' is an access or acupressure point at various points along the meridians. There are many of these tsubos or access points just under the skin, along each of the twelve major meridians. Stimulating these points with finger or elbow pressure can remove the stagnant Qi that collects in the tsubos, thereby helping to balance the flow of energy throughout the body. Accurate location of the tsubos will obviously enhance the effectiveness of the treatment. Fortunately, they are generally located at a weak spot on the body i.e. between muscle and bone or near the tip of a nerve and often in a slight depression or indentation on the body.

Reference to the charts will help identify the locations of the points used in the 20-minute sequence. The 12 major meridians have the following number of tsubos or acupressure points:

Lung	11
Large Intestine	20
Stomach	45
Spleen	21
Heart	9
Small Intestine	19
Bladder	67
Kidney	27
Gall Bladder	44
Liver	14
Heart Protector	9
Triple Heater	23
Conception Vessel	24
Governing Vessel	28

There are eight extraordinary Vessels or pathways, connecting and collecting Qi which are not directly linked to organ systems but transfer

THE TWELVE MAJOR MERIDIANS AND TWO EXTRAORDINARY VESSELS

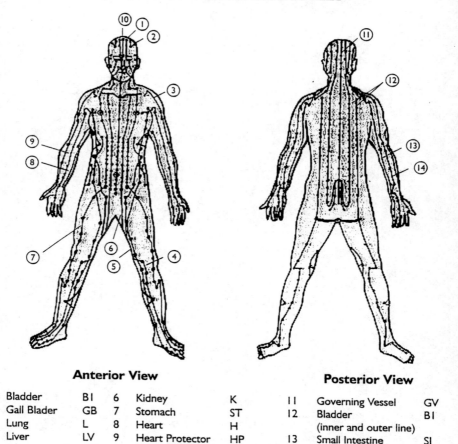

Anterior View   **Posterior View**

1	Bladder	BI	6	Kidney	K	11	Governing Vessel	GV
2	Gall Blader	GB	7	Stomach	ST	12	Bladder	BI
3	Lung	L	8	Heart	H		(inner and outer line)	
4	Liver	LV	9	Heart Protector	HP	13	Small Intestine	SI
5	Spleen	SP	10	Conception Vessel	CV	14	Triple Heater	TH

Editorial omission from p28

The Metal Element
The Lung Acupressure Points LU 1 – 11

This meridian governs the intake of pure Qi, eliminates impure Qi and is related to grief. Influences the descent of Qi to the kidneys and the production of urine.

Yin – Starts in the space between the first and second rib near the shoulder and ends on the outside edge of the thumb at the base of the nail.

The Large Intestine Meridian Acupressure Points LI 1 – 20

Supports the function of the small intestine and absorbs water.

Yang – Starts on the outer edge of the index finger at the base of the nail and runs along the arm to the face ending at the outside edge of the nostril.

energy to the major meridians as needed. The two most well known of these are the Governing Vessel and the Conception Vessel.

During a seated acupressure massage session, especially if the legs are included, dozens of acupressure points on all the major meridians are stimulated to help balance the flow of energy throughout the body.

THE TWELVE MAJOR MERIDIANS AND TWO EXTRAORDINARY VESSELS

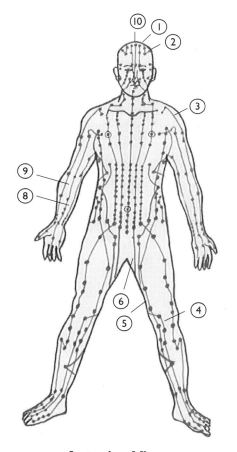

Anterior View

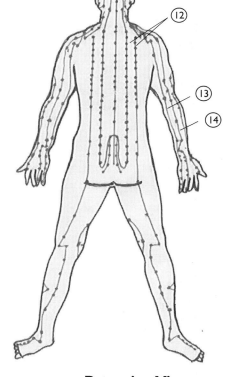

Posterior View

1	Bladder	Bl	7	Stomach	ST
2	Gall Bladder	GB	8	Heart	H
3	Lung	L	9	Heart Protector	HP
4	Liver	LV	10	Conception Vessel	CV
5	Spleen	SP			

11	Governing Vessel	GV
12	Bladder	Bl
	(inner and outer line)	
13	Small Intestine	SI
14	Triple Heater	TW

Quick Reference Notes for the Twelve Major Meridians and Two Extraordinary Vessels

The Two Extraordinary Vessels

They act as reservoirs of Qi for the twelve major meridians, filling and emptying as required.

Conception Vessel (Ren) Acupressure Points CV 1-24

Yin – Starts midway between the anus and the genitals, runs in a straight line up the front of the body and ends at the midline below the lower lip.

Governing Vessel (Du) Acupressure Points GV 1-28

Yang – Starts midway between the coccyx and the anus and runs straight up the midline of the back, over the head and ends on the inside of the mouth at the junction of the gum and upper lip.

The Water Element

Bladder Meridian Acupressure Points BL 1-67

The Bladder meridian is the longest meridian in the body. Some of the bladder acupressure points on the back, Shu points, have direct energy links with other meridians or organ systems, all of which are stimulated during the seated acupressure massage sequence.

Yang – Starts on the inner corner of the eye and ends on the outer edge of the little toe.

Kidney Meridian Acupressure Points K 1-27

The kidney meridian and the bladder meridian are paired or sister meridians.

Yin – Starts on the sole of the foot and ends in the depression on the lower edge of the collar bone, two thumb widths from the midline.

The Wood Element

The Liver Meridian Acupressure Points LV1-14

The liver meridian moves Qi through the body and is related to anger.

Yin – Starts on the inner margin of the big toe at the base of the nail and ends between the 6th and 7th ribs, just below the nipple.

The Gall Bladder Meridian Acupressure Points GB1-44
Related to storage of bile, and affects tendons.

Yang – Starts in the small depression at the outer corner of the eye and ends at the outer edge of the little toe at the base of the nail.

The Fire Element

The Heart Meridian Acupressure Points H 1-9
Controls the transformation of food Qi into blood and is related to joy.

Yin – Starts in the centre of the armpit and ends on the base of the little finger on the inside edge.

The Small Intestine Meridian Acupressure Points SI 1-19
Treats pains in shoulder, back, neck, wrists and elbow, related to digestion and body fluids.

Yang – Starts at the outer edge of the little finger at the base of the nail and ends in front of the small piece of cartilage that forms the front part of the ear.

Heart Protector (Pericardium Meridian) Acupressure Points HP1-9
Has a similar function to the heart and pressing points can reduce vomiting and nausea.

Yin – Starts on the chest on the lateral side of the nipple in the space between the 4th and 5th ribs and ends at the centre on the tip of the middle finger.

The Triple Heater (Sanjiao) Meridian Acupressure Points TH 1-23
This meridian supports the pericardium and regulates the body fluids.

Yang – Starts at the outside of the fourth finger at the base of the nail and ends on the outside tip of the eyebrow.

The Earth Element

The Spleen Meridian Acupressure Points SP1-21

This meridian governs Qi centrally and to the extremities and is related to worry.

Yin – Starts on the outer edge of the big toe at the base of the nail and ends 6 thumb widths below the armpit, between the 6th and 7th ribs.

The Stomach Meridian Acupressure Points ST 1-45

Separates essence from food and sends them to the spleen and small intestine.

Yang – Starts just above lower edge of the eye socket in line with the pupil and ends on the outside edge of the second toe at the base of the nail.

Chapter 3
Stress in the Workplace

Is the boss a Sabre-toothed Tiger?

Every era in the history of mankind has created different types of stress. Our early ancestors were mostly concerned with basic survival, finding food and shelter and fighting off predators. Facing a sabre-toothed tiger would certainly raise the stress profiles of the times, but at least the denizens of the caves could burn off the adrenalin and other stress hormones, either by running like the wind or by holding their ground and fighting for their lives.

Some stress is vital for our survival, otherwise we would not bother to get up in the morning. However, most people will agree that the advent of information technology and all the spin-offs from industry have pushed the vast majority of the working population into a state of constant high biochemical stress, with inadequate in-house strategies for ameliorating it. The result of some of these developments is measurable in a survey published in July 2000 by the Confederation of British Industry in conjunction with PPP. Statistics from the CBI Focus on Absence Survey indicate that the cost to British Industry due to absence from work is £10.5 billion, with an average number of 7.8 days per worker lost due to absence. In fairness, it is worth noting that there has been an improvement since the 1999 survey when the average number of lost days was 8.5. Are we beginning to see an impact from the growing numbers of companies who have introduced various stress management programmes?

A quick troll through the Internet revealed 92,000 sites dealing with stress management in the workplace. The scientific and medical journals and the press have been devoting a lot of space publishing Government and privately funded research and surveys relating to work-related upper limb disorders (WRULD), computer vision syndrome (CVS) and other manifestations of stress-related illnesses. Clearly, a whole new industry in stress management is developing in response to the demand.

Stress Specifics

The stress word is bandied about quite freely these days. We talk about being 'stressed out,' and most people have daily experiences that are major causes of stress, such as a near-miss experience on the motorway on the way to work, or an agitated boss looking for sales figures. It is worthwhile reviewing the various causes and manifestations of stress both physiological and psychological, that clients may present with.

'Hard work never killed anyone' our grandparents were wont to say and that is probably true as long as we can respect the cycle of our ultradian rhythms. It has been established that we all need a short break from any routine task every 90 minutes to stay healthy. In the office environment, sitting non-stop at a computer, possibly under flickering artificial light that throws glare and reflections onto the screen, and having lunch at the desk, is probably one of the quickest and most common routes to stress-related illness.

Someone once said that stress is more of an inner problem than an outer problem. In other words, how we deal with the stressful situation is more important than the situation itself. The psychologists have identified two basic personality types:

1. Type A is prone to high levels of stress, being impatient, uptight and highly driven and frequently set high goals for themselves and others.
2. Type B is calm, reasonable and more laid back. Most people will have some qualities from both type A and B but recognition of which type predominates may help to assess their stress triggers.

Holmes – Rahe Stress Scale

This scale grades life's events and changes according to the amount of stress they cause. If you have experienced changes giving you a total of over 50 in the last 6-12 months, then you may be experiencing some degree of stress:

1. Death of someone close   100
2. Divorce/separation   75
3. Separation   65
4. Injury/illness   53
5. Marriage   50
6. Redundancy/fired   47
7. Retirement   45
8. Pregnancy   40
9. Birth of a child   39
10. Change in finances   38
11. Argument with spouse   35
12. Child leaving home   29
13. Trouble with in-laws   29
14. Completing education   27
15. Trouble with boss   23
16. Change of work   20
17. Moving house   16
18. Going on holiday   15
19. Christmas   12
20. Breaking the law   11

Environmental factors too, contribute to stress levels, electromagnetic radiation from computer screens, artificial lighting, poor workplace ergonomics, noise, traffic pollution and overcrowding all take their toll. Needless to say, too many cups of tea and coffee, cigarettes, sugar and salt also create stress reactions, including increased output of stress hormones, nervous tension and fatigue.

What happens to the body during a stress reaction?

When faced with a challenge, the body responds biochemically in a way unchanged since the dawn of mankind. The reactions involve the brain, the nervous system and virtually every part of the body. There is an instant increase in the flow of adrenaline, cortisol and noradrenalin. Adrenaline speeds up the heart and respiration rate and increases muscle tension. Noradrenalin and cortisol create a feeling of excitement by raising blood sugar levels for quick thinking and for the extra energy needed to deal with conflict. Thyroxin stimulates the body to react quickly and endorphins act as natural painkillers. The digestive system contracts, the skin sweats and the mouth turns dry. These are all autonomic responses of the fight or flight mechanism and cannot be controlled voluntarily. This is great when the cause of the challenge is the tiger, or even when white water rafting. However, when this occurs in modern commercial life, the stress challenges may happen several times in one day. If there is no acceptable way to fight or run or to burn off the excessive secretion of hormones, people are left feeling tired, irritable, anxious, frustrated and susceptible to illness and infections. Medical research has shown that there are stress-related links to a number of serious and potentially serious conditions including:

- Cardiovascular ailments including high blood pressure, angina and coronary disease.
- Cancer.
- Strokes.
- Digestive problems such as irritable bowel syndrome, colitis and stomach ulcers.
- Asthma and allergies including eczema and psoriasis.
- Diabetes.
- Depression.
- Alcohol abuse.
- Computer Vision Syndrome (CVS) and other Repetitive Strain Injuries (RSI).

Apart from the personal misery caused by all of the above conditions, lost working days run into millions, and for a large corporate company, losing a single top executive to a stress-related illness can cost hundreds or thousands of pounds.

The more high-profile debilitating conditions such as repetitive strain injury and computer vision syndrome alone, are costing millions in litigation fees in the US, Canada and more recently in the UK.

Repetitive Strain Injuries (RSI)

What is commonly referred to as repetitive strain injury is not just a modern phenomenon or confined to keyboard users. Before the Industrial

Revolution, 18th century scribes and notaries suffered from wrist tenosynovitis (inflammation of the tendons and surrounding sheaths, often caused by repeated strain or trauma). By the end of the 18th century, machines had taken over and the occurrence of RSI symptoms in workers was reduced. In the 19th century, the most frequently recorded sufferers were musicians and tennis players.

Today, RSI symptoms have been reported as affecting people across the board of modern working life. The main factors that can contribute to RSI are:

- Static and incorrect posture.
- Overuse.
- Working long hours.
- Previous injuries in muscles and tendons.
- Exposure to cold.
- Dissatisfaction with your job and stress.

Workers who are particularly RSI prone include:

- Keyboard operators.
- Bank clerks.
- Switchboard operators.
- Supermarket cashiers.
- Waiters.
- Housepainters.
- Assembly line workers.
- Seamstresses.
- Hairdressers.
- Manual labourers.
- Children too, are beginning to show signs of the condition with the repeated use of the keyboard for computer games.

In the target-driven competitive environments of most modern workplaces, it is easy to see how people fall into the trap of over-riding the warning signs the body gives out, such as fatigue, tired eyes, aches and stiffness in joints and muscles. A classic example would be the keyboard worker sitting for hours in front of a computer screen with wrists flexed, elbows bent and shoulders hunched, using only minimal finger movements. This activity or lack of it, will eventually compress the median nerve, possibly at various points along its course from the brachial plexus to the fingers, and possibly lead to a painful condition referred to as Carpal Tunnel Syndrome (CTS). Anderseon et al 1994 define the condition as, 'a common painful disorder of the wrist and hand induced by compression on the median nerve between the inelastic carpal ligament and other structures within the carpal tunnel'.

Practitioners can test to see if the client has CTS by applying Phalen's Test. The client places both elbows on the table with vertical forearms and wrists flexed. If the client experiences numbness and tingling within 60 seconds along the pathway of the median nerve to the thumb and fingers, the test is positive.

CARPAL TUNNEL SYNDROME

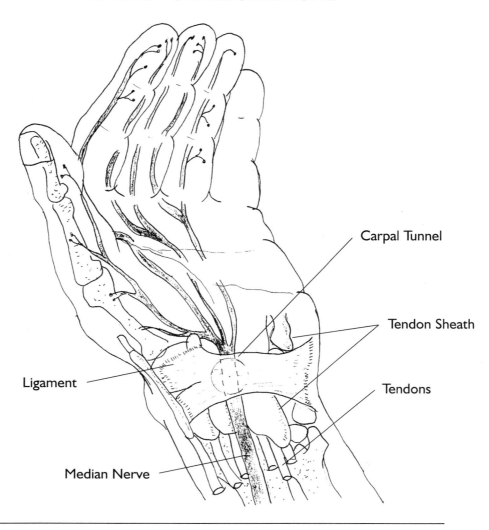

Carpal Tunnel

Tendon Sheath

Ligament

Tendons

Median Nerve

During the basic 20-minute seated acupressure massage sequence, the median nerve pathway is worked on, and this will help to relieve symptoms of CTS. However, the practitioner can spend longer working on this problem with the additional techniques that are taught specifically to relieve this condition. These techniques are described in a later chapter.

In 1988, to meet the public demand for information and help, the RSI Association, a registered charity with its head office in London, was set up to support people concerned about Carpal Tunnel Syndrome, and other RSI illnesses. Their mission statement is:

"The RSI Association is working towards a world in which the dangers of contracting RSI are fully recognised, where the risks are minimised and prevention is seen as a priority where accurate diagnosis, effective treatment and rehabilitation are prompt, and where no-one suffers long-term illness because of RSI."

There are however, more and more cases of claims going through the Courts. On 9th April 2000, a young woman in her twenties was awarded record damages of £243,792 against Barclays Bank PLC. She had developed a type of CTS (De Quervain's tenovaginitis) that caused excruciating pain in the thumb and restricted movement. Proper workplace assessment, and regular breaks from the computer screen with some stretching and movement, would in all probability, have prevented her condition.

The RSI Association is a good resource for practitioners wanting to gather the latest statistics and research into the impact of upper limb disorders in the workplace. They publish a monthly newsletter with current information from the Health and Safety Executive, the Trade Union Council, The Department for Education and Employment together with the latest relevant research from the scientific press. There are many excellent books and information on the Internet offering guidance on the prevention of RSI (see recommended further reading).

Computer Vision Syndrome (CVS)

Another work-related injury that is receiving attention in the scientific journals and in the Courts, is Computer Vision Syndrome. Operators who use a computer screen for more than two hours every day, may experience symptoms now classified as Computer Vision Syndrome. Symptoms include:

- Eye irritations such as red, itchy or watery eyes.
- Tired eyes.
- Difficulty in focusing.
- Headaches.
- Backaches.
- Muscle spasms.

A decade ago, a Ministry of Defence spokesman was moved to comment that, 'Eye problems are more than doubled with heavy computer use.' (Dodd, 1990). In America today, some 60 million people are suffering from eye problems due to computer work, with a million new cases being reported every year.

The human eye was not designed for staring at a computer screen. The image on the screen is made up of thousands of pixels or tiny dots and the eye is constantly trying to focus and make sense of these tiny images and the eye muscles for accommodation become tired. Also, with prolonged use and intense concentration on the project on the screen, people forget to blink as often, and the eyes dry out and become sore. Tests have proven that when working on a computer, individuals blink at less than half their normal rate. This in turn makes it more difficult to focus, causing blurred vision and possibly headaches and neck pain. To compound this problem, artificial lighting can cause glare and reflection on the screens. Not too many modern offices have adequate windows with far-reaching views of green fields and hills to give tired, sore eyes a much-needed visual break.

A report from the Journal of the American Optometric Association ranks the symptoms of CVS in order of their frequency:

1. Eyestrain (sore or fatigued eyes).
2. Headache.
3. Slowness in changing focusing distance.
4. Blurred vision after close-up work.
5. Eye irritation (burning, dryness, redness).
6. Contact lens discomfort.
7. Neck, back and shoulder pain due to poor posture.

According to the National Institute of Occupational Safety and Health, (USA), Computer Vision Syndrome is the number one cause of eyestrain in the workplace. The symptoms are severe enough to cause productivity problems, increased error rates, dissatisfaction with the job, absenteeism and potential health insurance and disability issues. In a recent survey of computer executives 86% reported symptoms of CVS after two or more hours of computer use.

As with Carpal Tunnel Syndrome and other upper limb disorders, Computer Vision Syndrome can be avoided if sensible preventative action is taken. Practitioners should advise clients who use computers for more than two hours every day to practice the following good habits:

- Make sure the computer screen is 20 – 24 inches from your eyes at about 20 degrees below eye level.

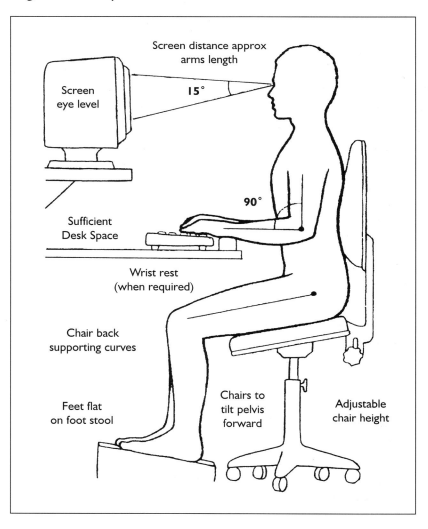

- If you use a document holder, keep it close to the screen.
- Dim the overhead lights and keep desk lamps low and properly adjusted so the light does not enter your eyes or fall on the screen.
- Shifting. Every 15 minutes, focus on distant objects to relax your eye muscles.
- Palm your eyes. Rub your hands together to create heat. Lean your elbows on a table and gently cup your eyes without pressing your hands into your eyes. Close your eyes and breathe deeply and slowly, visualising that you are looking into blackness. This creates a profound relaxation of the internal and external muscles of the eyes (it quietens the mind too).
- Blink frequently to lubricate and sweep the eye clear of dust particles.
- Get into natural light as much as possible.

No Light at Night (Nolan)

Another little-known issue that affects physical and mental health, is the importance of sleeping in total darkness at night to optimise the production of melatonin. Melatonin is a cancer preventing hormone that helps you sleep and also contributes to the timing of the biological clock of the body. The effects of artificial light on the brain at night can be detrimental to your health (Silk, 1999). The eyelids, even when closed, are translucent and allow waves of photic stimulation to travel deep into the pineal gland in the brain. The illuminated faces of bedside clocks, red charge lights from bedside phones, TV and computer screen left on standby during the hours of sleep, and light from street lamps and children's night-lights, will enter the eye through the closed lids, strike the retina and stimulate the photoreceptors. The chemical chain reaction continues, ultimately inhibiting the production of melatonin by the cells of the pineal gland. This could in part lead to hyperactivity in children and severely disrupted sleep patterns in adults with possible severe mood swings and behavioural changes. Once again a few simple strategies can help prevent light at night entering the eyes:

- Cover the windows with dark, lined curtains or blinds to cut out the light from street lamps.
- Switch off computers and TVs in the bedroom at night when sleeping.
- Cover clock faces and phone chargers with a scarf.
- Shut the bedroom door and cover the cracks if a light is left on in the hallway.

- Train small children to sleep without a night-light.
- If none of the above is possible, wear an eye mask like the ones they hand out on aircraft.

This overview of 20th century stress, with the alarming impact that stress-related illnesses has, not only on industry but also on the health and well-being of millions of people in the workforce, underscores the valuable rôle that practitioners of seated acupressure massage can play both in private practice and in the workplace.

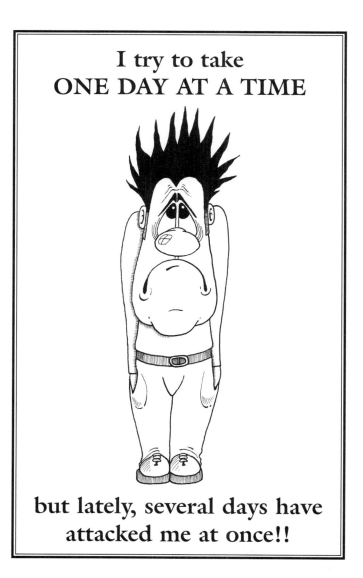

Chapter 4

Why Seated Acupressure Massage is the Ideal Therapy for the Modern Practitioner

There is no doubt that many employers are responding to the wake-up call from staff members demanding a better working environment. Human Resources departments are awash with new legislation designed to protect the employee from discrimination, unfair dismissal, and the right to sue if they sustain a work-related personal injury. Consultants are brought in to run Positive Personal Development and Stress Management Seminars and advice is taken on Strategies for Compliance with EC Legislation and Litigation. Some employers are bringing in Feng Shui consultants to improve the energy flow in their building. The IT industry in particular is fiercely competitive and employers go to great lengths to keep their staff, by providing them with the latest upgrades in WAP mobile phones and high performance cars. One well-known IT company spends a thousand pounds every Friday afternoon buying in potato crisps, beer and wine for the staff's 'happy hour' – but, was unwilling to budget for weekly seated acupressure massage sessions (maximum cost £280) for a handful of their most stressed employees! Some large companies have on-site fitness centres, counselling services and Occupational Health Departments where nurses and a physiotherapist are on hand to treat sick and injured employees. The counsellors, nurses and physiotherapists all do a great job, but their work is reactive, as employees normally wait until a problem is debilitating before they make an appointment to be seen.

Fortunately, more and more enlightened employers are beginning to recognise the benefits of a direct 'hands-on' approach, and are allowing staff members to receive massage sessions 'on-site' during working hours. Employees perceive this as a positive commitment of management for their wellbeing, and staff morale rises accordingly.

Almost any type of kindly touch has therapeutic value and the physical and psychological benefits of massage in particular are well documented. Practitioners of table massage are well aware of the vulnerability some people experience when they have to remove most of their clothing and lie down to receive a treatment. Even offering Reflexology, as wonderful as it is, can inhibit people as they often have major issues about the shape or odour of their feet.

What are the benefits of Seated Acupressure Massage?

It is easy to see why seated acupressure massage has become the treatment of choice for the workplace. It is quick, effective, clothes stay on, no messy oils are used, the massage chair is comfortable and supports the whole body, and afterwards the employee is relaxed, alert and ready to get back to work. People who would otherwise never consider having a massage because they are inhibited, too busy or just plain sceptical, are quite happy to jump on the massage chair in the familiar surroundings of their own office building or gym. You can see the client's body visibly relaxing as the chair takes the strain off the spine and you encourage them to take a few deep breaths. (Shallow breathing is another symptom of stress).

Unlike the effleurage strokes of body massage, seated acupressure massage works directly on the 12 major meridians and their associated organs and systems, balancing the flow of Qi or energy round the whole body. As a result, the tension in tight muscles and joints is eased, the circulation of the blood and lymph improves and the immune, endocrine and nervous systems all benefit from the unblocking of stagnant energy in the acupressure points. The rhythm of the 20 minutes of formalised moves, the Kata, promotes a sense of wellbeing in the client, leaving them calm and clearly focused, but more importantly, ready to tackle the rest of the working day with renewed enthusiasm! To summarise, a 20-minute seated acupressure massage treatment will have the following effects:

- Relaxing and calming of the nervous system.
- A decrease in blood pressure and pulse.
- Relaxation of tight and sore muscles.
- Dispersal of toxins.
- Release of stagnant energy.
- Improved circulation of the lymphatic system, which strengthens the immune system.
- Improved alertness and concentration.

Consequently, there are many common conditions that will respond to and improve with seated acupressure massage sessions. The list is long, but some of the most common stress-related ailments that practitioners encounter either in the workplace or in private practice include:

- Anxiety and depression.
- Backache and sciatic pain.
- Repetitive strain injuries such as carpal tunnel syndrome or frozen shoulder.
- Asthma and other breathing difficulties.
- Sinus problems.
- Eyestrain.
- Headaches/migraines.
- Insomnia.
- Chronic fatigue syndrome.
- Menstrual tension.
- Stress related muscle tension.
- Skin problems.
- High blood pressure * (see contraindications).

Screening the Client

As with any other complementary therapy, a full medical history should be taken before starting the treatment. Make sure that the screening is carried out in such a way that any potential problems are uncovered and discussed.

Use your experience and powers of observation to help you ascertain if they are able to receive a massage. Even if your client is booked in for a series of treatments and you are familiar with their medical history, it is important to carry out a minimum screening to cover each session. Also at health exhibitions, charity events or corporate demonstrations when you may only have a short time with a client, the basic screening questions need to be asked and a disclaimer form signed by the client.

The following areas are either contraindicated or where special care must be taken, and the sequence modified accordingly.

Contraindications and 'Special Care' Conditions

- Women who are pregnant or trying to conceive should not receive any acupressure point work. Modify the massage work on the chair using some of the table massage effleurage – type strokes. It will still feel wonderful on the back, neck, arms, hands and head.
- People with high or low blood pressure may suddenly feel light-headed and faint. It is best not to work on people who are on medication to reduce high blood pressure, as this may lower it too much. With permission and co-operation from the client's GP, it may be possible to have the client's BP monitored after treatments with the possible outcome of the medication being reduced if the blood pressure regulates naturally.
- If the client has a history of fainting, or has low blood sugar or low blood pressure, make sure they have had something to eat earlier that day. If their blood pressure is anything more than slightly low, check with their GP.
- People recovering from recent surgery or who have been seriously ill must have consent from their doctor.
- Do not work heavily on the lower back if the client has just had a large meal.
- Do not work on areas such as fractures, dislocations, and recent injections.
- Avoid treatment if the client has had alcohol or recreational drugs.
- Skin conditions such as psoriasis and eczema are not contraindicated if there is no broken skin – just avoid any friction moves. If the skin is broken, massage may still take place. However avoid the affected area. In infectious skin conditions, avoid contact.

- If the client has suffered an injury or trauma within twenty-four hours.
- Any communicable diseases such as influenza or tuberculosis.

Receive consent from their GP or SPECIALIST for the following conditions

- Epilepsy.
- Diabetes (they may have peripheral neuropathy).
- Cancer.
- Arthritis.
- Rheumatism.
- Osteoporosis.
- Osteoarthritis.
- Thrombosis.
- Hip or shoulder replacement surgery or metal plates in the body.
- If client is on medication.

At the end of the screening process, ask the client if there is anything else they may want to ask before starting the session.

What to do if the Client faints or feels faint

Remain calm – get the client to lie down in the recovery position, or place their head between their legs. Give the client a glass of water. Do not leave the client whilst they are feeling unwell. Reassure them and ascertain a likely reason they may have fainted – i.e. an empty stomach, recent illness, low blood pressure, medication?

Preparation

If you have an appointment set with a client, make sure you arrive in plenty of time to set up your chair. Ensure that the room is a good temperature and preferably in a quiet, private area. Your body and mind also need to prepare to work on a client and a few minutes of stretching, Tai Chi or "Do-In" (awakening the body by working on the meridians with a loose fist) are ideal ways to prepare.

Loosen and stretch the arms, hands and fingers too before you start working. Too many massage therapists have to give up their profession early because they develop painful hand conditions that could be avoided with a good hand-maintenance programme. The following self-massage routine is based on the suggestions of Japanese Anma master and teacher, Shogo Mochizuki, and is ideal not only for massage practitioners but for anyone, such as keyboard operators, who have to make lengthy repetitive movements with the hands and arms.

1. Warm the muscles of the arms and shoulders with vigorous friction rubs and squeezes. Rotate the shoulders in both directions.
2. Place your arm on the table with your palm upwards. With the heel of your other hand on the medial border of the forearm, firmly squeeze and rotate the muscles of the forearm until they are warm and loose.
3. Percuss the length of the forearm with a loose fist or with the back of your other hand.
4. With your opposite thumb rotate the muscles of the wrist starting at the thenar side of the carpal bones (on the lung meridian). Apply the rotation by moving the whole hand, not just the thumb, and work your way round the wrist until you arrive back where you started.
5. Stroke firmly with the opposite thumb down the length of all spaces between the metacarpal bones from the wrist to the base of the fingers, back and front of the hand. Massage, squeeze and rotate the fingers of each hand with the thumb and index finger of the opposite hand.

Explaining the Massage to a new Client

If it is the first time with a new client, an introduction and even a brief description of the massage and some reassurance may be necessary. Some people may not have had any sort of massage before and may be slightly apprehensive. Don't be tempted to go into a long description about Yin and Yang and the Five Element Theory. If it is their first time, they are probably there more for the experience of the massage, so keep the explanation simple. Show them how to sit in the chair, explain that they do not have to remove clothes and that no oils will be used. For their first treatment, most people are happy to hear that the massage will make them feel better by relieving tension and stiffness in the back and neck and that they should feel more relaxed but energised and clear-headed. During subsequent treatments, you can introduce more specific information about the effects of acupressure massage if it seems appropriate for your client. Demonstrate how to sit in the chair and ensure the client will be comfortable – i.e. they have removed ties, belts, glasses, watches or items of jewellery if necessary and loosened collars. Treat personal effects respectfully and place them nearby and make sure the client does not leave without them at the end of the session.

Screening

Ensure that you carry out the minimum screening, or take client notes. This is not only essential to ensure that the client is not contraindicated in any way, but complete notes will provide you with specific treatment details and feedback over a period of time.

Hygiene and Appearance

Ensure that you have a professional appearance, that your hands are clean, fingernails short and long hair tied back. It is not sensible or practical to wear white trousers or a white skirt or dress to give seated acupressure massage. A white cotton top and dark, loose-fitting comfortable trousers always look smart and professional. If you have badges from your training school and organization for complementary therapists such as the Guild of Complementary Practitioners, then wear them. You earned them through your hard work and it shows your client that you are a qualified professional. Some practitioners like to work in bare feet – this is acceptable in private practice but is not recommended in the workplace. Wear white or dark trainers or mules that are soft enough to let you shuffle back on the ball of your foot without the shoe slipping off your foot or cutting off the circulation.

Clean the chair and face rest after each client (in front of them) and wash your hands. Some practitioners like to use paper or towelling face covers on their chairs. If you choose not to use face covers, have a box of man-sized tissues handy in case your client is sensitive to the vinyl or leather, sweats a lot, or wears heavy make-up.

Music and aromatherapy burners are sometimes appropriate, obviously depending on the venue, but be careful of your choice of oils, nothing too heady. Choose light, uplifting oils such as mandarin, lavender or peppermint.

Client Comfort

Remain aware of body language – some clients may not want to tell you if they are experiencing discomfort. Check that the pressure is comfortable, especially when using elbow pressure on the back and thumb pressure around the occipital base. Ensure that they tell you at any time if they would like you to alter the pressure. The first line of pressure can be used to warm the area whilst the second can go slightly deeper.

Practitioner Posture

Maintain a correct posture at all times, bending at the hips, not the waist. Use your body weight to apply pressure and stay relaxed – you will not tire yourself out as much and the pressure will be much more even. Maintain contact with the client at all times and gently apply and release pressure. Breathe from your Hara (centre just below your navel). Keep yourself grounded, letting the energy flow through your body and in turn, the movements will flow better.

Water for Practitioner and Client

Advise the client to drink a large glass of still water after the massage. This is to flush any toxins that may have been released from the muscles into the blood stream and prevent stiffness (as they would if they had taken part in any sort of exercise). It is also very important that you, the practitioner, drink a glass of still water after each client to re-hydrate and to keep your energy levels up.

Chapter 5
Seated Acupressure Massage Sequence

This chapter gives a detailed step-by-step guide for practitioners who have trained or are undergoing training in seated acupressure massage. For easy assimilation during practice sessions, the instructions are simple without too many references to the precise anatomical position of the points. More detailed descriptions can be found under the photographs of the sequence elsewhere in this chapter and from the charts.

Centre

Before you start work on any client, take some time to centre yourself. This allows you to become more focused and grounded. Once the client is in the chair, place your hands on their shoulders and ask them to take a deep breath and drop their shoulders. Brush down the back twice, then run your thumbs down either side of the spine lightly and slowly, taking the opportunity to check for any curvature and muscle tension.

Double Palm Press: *(five positions, twice)*

Place one foot behind the chair, front knee slightly bent and the other straight on the ball of the foot ready to shuffle back between each pressure. Place your hands on either side of the spine, arms straight. Ask your client to take a deep breath and continue breathing deeply and evenly. Flex your front knee and allow your body weight to transfer itself through your arms to the client's back as they breathe out. The pressure should be at 90 degrees to the client, with downward pressure for the last position.

This is the first firm contact with the client. It gets them used to your touch, opens the back for further work and encourages deep breathing.

Archer Press: *(three positions, twice)*

Stepping round to the side, place the left foot in front and keep the back leg straight. Place the heel of your right palm on the erector spinae muscles, fingers pointing away from you and resting gently over the spine and your

UPPER BACK
Nine Points, Four Scapula Points and Three Trapezius Points

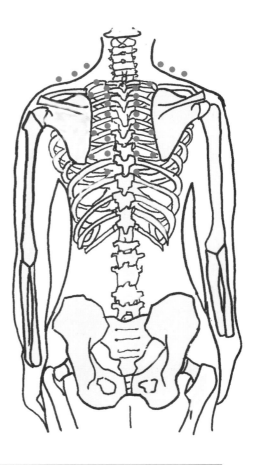

Upper Back
Small Intestine and Bladder Meridian
Thoracic spine T1 – T10

1. SI 15
2. BL 11
3. BL 12
4. BL 13
5. BL 14
6. BL 15
7. BL 16
8. BL 17
9. BL 18

Four Scapula Points
Small Intestine and Bladder Meridians
In line with medial border of scapula

1. SI 13
2. BL 37
3. BL 39
4. BL 41

Three Trapezius Points
Gall Bladder and Large Intestine Meridian
Starts close to neck and shoulder, ends behind acromion process

1. Nameless
2. GB 21
3. LI 16

left hand on the client's shoulder. Looking straight ahead, with shoulders facing forwards, flex your left knee, pulling the muscle away from the spine and gradually increasing the pressure.

Forearm Press: *(three positions, twice)*

Keeping your left hand on the shoulder, place the underside of your right forearm at the junction of the neck and shoulder. Let your body weight sink into three points across the top of the trapezius, remaining on the muscle. This move should be slow in both applying the pressure and releasing.

Erector Spinae: *(nine points, twice)*

Place your right leg in line behind the client's spine and stand on the ball of the right foot. Position the elbow in point 1, located about one inch away from the spine between C7 and T1. Relax the wrist keeping the elbow at right angles to the client's back. As the elbow bends, allow the pressure to sink gradually into the point, by bending your front knee. Come in half an inch closer to the spine for points 2 to 9, which lie in the spaces between the vertebrae. Shuffle your back foot back between points. Ensure you do not apply any pressure directly to the spine.

Scapula Medial Border: (Elbow Work) *(four points, twice)*

Start half an inch to the right of the superior medial border of the scapula roughly opposite T1 and work down 4 points in a straight line, approximately one and a half inches apart. The last point should be level with the bottom of the scapula.

Trapezius Crest: *(three positions, twice)*

Elbow on trapezius crest close to neck. Allow the elbow to sink into the first point, moving outwards. Point 3 is in the triangle formed by the clavicle and the spine of the scapula.

Scapula to Sacrum Rub and Brush Down

Using the heel of the right hand, rub in a vigorous circular motion on the erector spinae muscles, from the shoulder to sacrum. Brush down.

Left Arm

Kneel or squat as you lower the client's arm giving it a gentle downward pull. Hold the top of the arm with both hands and rub down to the wrist twice. Starting at the top of the arm squeeze the muscles with both hands in 5 positions ending at the wrist.

I. Deltoid to Elbow:
(five points, twice)

Locate point 1 which is in the slight depression at the top of the arm in the deltoid muscle. With your thumbs, using a hand over hand technique work down 5 equidistant points ending above the elbow in line with the client's middle finger.

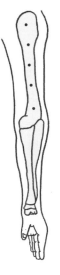

Posterior Upper Arm
Large Intestine Meridian

1. Nameless
2. LI 14
3. Nameless
4. Nameless
5. Nameless

The squeezing and vibration on upper arm also stimulates the small intestine and triple heater meridians.

Posterior Lower Left Arm
(five points, twice)

2. Large Intestine Meridian:
(five points, twice)

Turn the hand so that the thumb is facing you. Using your right thumb, locate Point 1 on the radius just below the elbow crease. Apply pressure in five positions ending on point 5 in the indentation on the wrist.

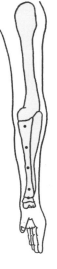

Posterior Lower Arm Large Intestine Meridian

1. LI 11
2. LI 9
3. LI 7
4. Nameless
5. LI 5
6. LI 4 (Great Eliminator)

Starts below elbow crease in line with the radius to the thumb

3. Triple Heater Meridian:
(five points, twice)

Turn the hand so that the back of the hand is facing you. Starting just below the elbow, apply pressure to five points between the radius and ulna using alternate hands. End on the wrist.

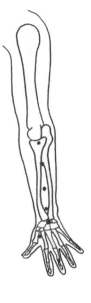

Posterior Lower Arm Triple Heater Meridian

1. Nameless
2. TH9
3. Nameless
4. TH5
5. TH4

Starts below elbow crease between radius and ulna in line with the middle finger

4. Small Intestine Meridian:
(five points, twice)

Turn the hand so the little finger is facing you. Using your left thumb, start just below the elbow and in the groove behind the ulna. Work down in five positions, finishing at the end of the ulna bone at the side of the wrist.

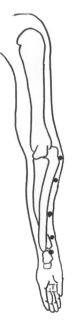

Posterior Lower Arm Small Intestine Meridian

1. SI 8
2. Nameless
3. SI 7
4. SI 6
5. SI 5

Starts below elbow crease behind ulna in line with the little finger

Wrist Squeeze

Squeeze the sides of the wrist twice with your thumb and forefinger as you walk around to the front. Place the arm back on the rest.

Hand Spread

Using the heels of your hands, firmly spread the back of the client's hand.

Thumb Strokes and Mobilisation

Stroke twice firmly down the back of the hand between the outer metacarpals, turning your thumbs towards you and finishing between the fingers. Follow with two firm jiggles, once again ending through the fingers. Repeat thumb strokes and jiggles down the inner metacarpals.

Great Eliminator (LI 4)

Squeeze twice between the client's thumb and index finger for a few seconds and pull away.

ANTERIOR LEFT ARM AND INNER HAND
Heart, Heart Protector and Lung Meridian

Heart Meridian:
(five points, twice)

Turn the arm over, and with your right thumb press five points starting below the elbow on the inside of the arm and ending on the wrist.

Heart Protector:
(five points, twice)

Thumb pressures down five points starting in the middle of the arm just below the elbow and finishing in the middle of the wrist.

Lung Meridian:
(five points, twice)

Starting on the outside crease of the arm below the elbow, press five points ending at the wrist.

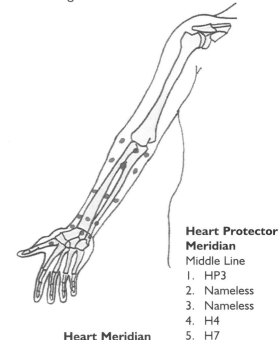

Heart Protector Meridian
Middle Line
1. HP3
2. Nameless
3. Nameless
4. H4
5. H7

Heart Meridian
In line with little finger. Starts just below the elbow crease, ends on wrist crease.
1. H3
2. Nameless
3. Nameless
4. H4
5. H7

Lung Meridian
In line with the thumb
1. L5
2. Nameless
3. L6
4. L7
5. L9
6. L10

Stroke Down

Stroke down twice from the elbow crease to the fingertips to open and relax the hand.

Tendon and Hand Spread

Using the heels of your hands spread open the palm.

Thumb Strokes and Mobilisation

Stroke twice firmly down the palm of the hand between the outer metacarpals, finishing between the fingers and repeat. Follow with two firm jiggles, once again ending through the fingers. Repeat thumb strokes and jiggles down the inner metacarpals.

Lung 10

Press lung 10 with your right thumb, located on the fleshy pad on the palm side of the thumb.

Coin Rub and Finger Clicks

Starting with the client's thumb, rub along the top and bottom and the sides of the thumb. Squeeze the edges of the nail and flick the energy away from your own body. Repeat for each of the fingers. Adopt a comfortable stance and make sure your back is straight.

Grasp Wrist and Extend Arm

Remain in contact with the client and keeping the arm under tension give a downward pull. Ask the client to breathe in and on the out breath stretch the arm up and slightly away from their body. You should be in a lunge position, facing forwards with your front knee bent. At full stretch, vibrate the hand. Gently lower the arm and squeeze the left shoulder with your left hand as you walk round in preparation for the Archer Press.

Right Upper Back and Shoulder

Archer Press: *(three positions, twice)*

Stepping round to the side, place the right foot in front and keep the back leg straight. Place the heel of your left palm on the erector spinae muscles, fingers resting gently over the spine and your right hand on the client's shoulder. Looking straight ahead, shoulders facing forwards, flex your right knee pulling the muscle away from the spine, gradually increasing the pressure.

Forearm Press: *(three positions, twice)*

Keeping your right hand on the shoulder, place the underside of your left forearm at the junction of the neck and shoulder. Let your body weight sink into three points across the top of the trapezius, remaining on the muscle. This move should be slow in both applying the pressure and releasing.

Elbow Work

Erector Spinae: *(nine points, twice)*

Place your left leg in line behind the client's spine and stand on the ball of the left foot. Position the elbow in point 1, located about one inch away from the spine between C7 and T1. Relax the wrist, keeping the elbow at right angles to the client's back. As the elbow bends, allow the pressure to sink gradually into the point by bending your front knee. Come in half an inch closer to the spine for points 2 to 9, which lie in the spaces between the vertebrae. Shuffle your back foot back between points. Ensure that you do not apply any pressure directly to the spine.

Scapula Medial Border: *(four points, twice)*

Start half an inch to the left of the superior medial border of the scapula roughly opposite T1 and work down 4 points in a straight line, approximately one and a half inches apart. The last point should be level with the bottom of the scapula.

Trapezius Crest: *(three positions, twice)*

Left elbow on the trapezius crest close to the neck. Allow the elbow to sink into the first point, moving outwards. Point 3 is in the triangle formed by the clavicle and the spine of the scapula.

Scapula to Sacrum Rub and Brush Down

Using the heel of the left hand, rub in a vigorous circular motion on the erector spinae muscles, from the shoulder to the sacrum. Brush down.

Right Arm

Kneel or squat as you lower the right arm, giving it a gentle downward pull. Hold the top of the arm with both hands and rub down to the wrist twice. Startimg at the top of the arm squeeze the muscles with both hands in 5 positions ending at the wrist. Repeat.

Deltoid to Elbow: *(five points, twice)*

Locate point 1 which is in the slight depression at the top of the arm in the deltoid muscle. With your thumbs, using a hand over hand technique work down 5 equidistant points ending above the elbow in line with the client's middle finger.

Posterior Lower Arm

Large Intestine Meridian: *(five points, twice)*

Turn the hand so that the thumb is facing you. Using your left thumb, locate Point 1 on the radius just below the elbow crease. Apply pressure in five positions ending on point 5 in the indentation on the wrist.

Triple Heater Meridian: *(five points, twice)*

Turn the hand so the back of the hand is facing you. Starting just below the elbow, apply pressure to five points between the radius and ulna using alternate hands. End on the wrist.

Small Intestine Meridian: *(five points, twice)*

Turn the hand so the little finger is facing you. Using your left thumb, start just below the elbow and in the groove behind the ulna. Work down in five positions, finishing at the side of the wrist.

Wrist Squeeze

Squeeze the sides of the wrist twice, with your thumb and forefinger as you walk around to the front. Place the arm back on the rest.

Hand Spread

Using the heels of your hands, firmly spread the back of the client's hand.

Thumb Strokes and Mobilisation

Stroke twice firmly down the back of the hand between the outer metacarpals, turning your thumbs towards you and finishing between the fingers. Follow with two firm jiggles, once again ending through the fingers. Repeat thumb strokes and jiggles down the inner metacarpals.

Great Eliminator: (LI 4)

Squeeze twice between the client's thumb and index finger for a few seconds and pull away.

Anterior Right Arm and Inner Hand

Heart Meridian: *(five points, twice)*

Turn the arm over, and with your left thumb, press five points starting below the elbow on the inside of the arm and ending on the wrist.

Heart Protector: *(five points, twice)*

Thumb pressures down five points starting in the middle of the arm just below the elbow and finishing in the middle of the wrist.

Lung Meridian: *(five points, twice)*

Starting on the outside crease of the arm below the elbow, press five points ending at the wrist. Stroke down twice to the fingertips to open and relax the hand.

Tendon and Hand Spread

Using the heels of your hands spread open the palm.

Thumb Strokes and Mobilisation

Stroke twice firmly and then jiggle down the palm of the hand between the outer metacarpals, finishing between the fingers and repeat. Repeat down the inner metacarpals.

Lung 10

Press lung 10 with the pad of your thumb, located on the fleshy area on the palm side of the thumb.

Coin Rub and Finger Clicks

Starting with the client's thumb, rub along the top and bottom and the sides of the thumb. Squeeze the edges of the nail, flicking the energy away. Repeat for each of the fingers.

Grasp Wrist and Extend Arm

Remain in contact with the client and keeping the arm under tension give a downward pull and ask the client to breathe in. On the out breath stretch the arm up and slightly away from their body. You should be in a lunge position, facing forwards with your front knee bent. At full stretch, vibrate the hand and gently lower the arm. Squeeze the right shoulder as you walk around to start the lower back.

LOWER BACK
Nine Points, Four Sacrum Points

Nine Points
Bladder Meridian from T10 – L5

1. BL 19
2. BL 20
3. BL 21
4. BL 22
5. BL 23
6. BL 24
7. BL 25
8. BL 26
9. BL 27
10. BL 28

Sacrum
Bladder Meridian from S1 – S4

1. BL 48
2. BL 29
3. BL 34
4. BL 35

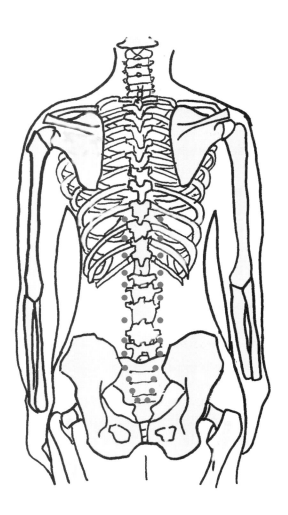

Double Palm Press *(five positions, twice)*

Brush down twice. Keeping your arms straight, front leg flexed at the knee and back leg on the ball of the foot. Your hands should be either side of the spine with fingers spread, starting just below the scapula. Ask the client to breathe deeply and on the out breath drop the weight in through your arms by bending your front knee.

Shuffle back with your back leg as you move down the spine. Work in five positions down the length of the lower back, ending at the sacrum. The last two pressures should have a downward intention.

Double Hand Butterfly Press: *(nine points, twice)*

Place your thumbs on either side of the spine between the 8th and 9th thoracic vertebrae. Flex your front knee and apply pressure into the point steadily and evenly. Work down nine positions to L5 in the intervertebral spaces. Continue to:

Sacrum Press: *(four points, twice)*

Using your thumbs, follow the shape of the sacrum starting at the outer edges and working inwards. Finish on point 4 just above the coccyx. This can help release lower back tension.

Gluteal Release

Squat or kneel behind the client. Using the heels of your hands with fingers pointing upwards, work in small circles from the sacrum outwards along the gluteus medius to the pelvic blade. Repeat the circles further down from the gluteus maximus to the hip joint. Stand up and brush down from shoulders to sacrum.

Neck and Scalp

Walk around to the left side.

Base of Skull

Place your left hand on the top of the client's head and ask them to look down to stretch the neck. Press up into the underside of the occipital base starting just left of centre, in five positions ending behind the mastoid process. Check the pressure and work gently on the last point as this can be very tender. Repeat.

OCCIPITAL BASE AND NECK
Three Trapezius Crest Points

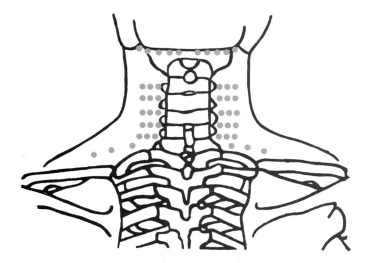

Occipital Base
Governing Vessel
and Gall Bladder

1. GV 16
2. Nameless
3. GB 20
4. Nameless
5. Nameless

**Three Trapezius
Crest Points**

Trigger Points

Neck Lines: *(three lines, five points each, twice)*

Place your right thumb close to the second cervical vertebrae with your fingers resting lightly on the opposite side of the neck. Work down in five positions twice, using the pad of the thumb to move the muscle away from the spine. Repeat for two more lines starting each line by moving about one fingers' width further from the spine. Work each line twice.

End Points From Neck Lines

These three points are found on the crest of the trapezius moving in towards C7. They are the ending points following the route of the three neck lines. Working on these points, two of which are also trigger points, can help release tension in the trapezius muscles and also helps move stagnant energy. Squeeze the left shoulder as you move round to the right side.

Base of Skull

Place your right hand on the top of the client's head and press up into the underside of the occipital base as before, starting just right of centre, in five positions ending behind the mastoid process. Repeat.

Neck Lines: *(three lines, five times each, twice)*

Place your left thumb close to the cervical vertebrae with your fingers resting lightly on the side of the neck. Start at the top of the neck and work down in five positions twice using the pad of the thumb to move the muscles away from the spine. Repeat this for two more lines, moving one finger's width away from the spine for each line. Work each line twice.

End Points From Neck Lines

Apply pressure with the left thumb on three points on the trapezius crest moving in towards C7. Repeat. Squeeze the right shoulder as you move to the back of the client. Brush down twice. Ask the client to take a breath and slowly sit up with their arms by their sides. Gently hold the client's head above the ears to centre them. Give a gentle upward lift.

Neck Stretch

Stand directly behind the client with your feet hip width apart. Left forearm palm up on the left shoulder and right hand on either side of their left ear, elbow up. Ensure your forearm does not rest on the client's head. Ask the client to take a breath, rotating your forearm inwards as you press down the left shoulder, gently move the head to the right and hold for 7 seconds. Centre. Repeat on the other side.

Scalp Massage

With the pads of your fingers and thumbs, massage in small circles moving the scalp. Make sure you stay away from the temples as this can be painful.

Scalp Lifts

Using the pads of your fingers and thumbs, firmly and briskly, lift your hands off the scalp to stimulate the flow of blood to the head.

Cupped Percussion

Clasp your hands together keeping a pocket of air between them as this creates a cushion effect for the client. If you haven't perfected this yet, then work very gently! With your wrists and hands loose, start from the occipital base, just left of the centre line and move up to the front of the hairline at the forehead and around the crown. End by cupping down to the right of the centre line, bringing your hands off together at the occipital base.

Shoulders

Double Forearm Press

With feet apart and forearms on the client's shoulders close into the neck, palms up, ask the client to take a breath. As they breathe out, drop your weight down and in three positions, move to the edge of the shoulder rotating your forearms and repeat.

Thumb Squeeze Rotation

Squeeze and rotate thumbs along the trapezius followed by four positions down either side of the spine and repeat.

Trapezius Squeeze

Using the palms of your hands, gently squeeze and lift the trapezius in three positions to the shoulder and down the upper arms. Repeat.

Chicken Wing Stretch

Slide your hands down the client's arms, supporting their forearms, with their palms up. Ask them to take a breath and drop the head forward. As they breathe out, bring their arms back and up. Keep your own elbows out to the side to increase their stretch. When the stretch is enough, hold that position for seven seconds then gently lower, giving the arms a downward pull.

Full and Final Brush Down

Brush the client down three times by sweeping the hands from the crown to the sacrum followed by once down the arms.

Shoulder Lifts

Say to your client, "Take a deep breath, and when I drop your shoulder, exhale". Grasp the upper arms firmly and lift. Briskly throw the arms down, brushing off the shoulders between each breath. Do this twice and on the third breath, keep your arms up and go straight into the hacking.

Percussion

Loose Hacking

As the client's shoulders drop, begin the percussion either side of the spine and work across the shoulders. Keep the wrists loose and the fingers apart, hack down to the mid-back. Bend your knees, keeping your back straight. Percussion will stimulate the circulation and help energise the client. Work along the trapezius and down either side of the spine, back up and repeat.

Praying Hands

Starting on the left shoulder, close to the spine, sandwich your hands together keeping your fingers apart and loose. Raise your elbows outwards. Make sure you do not work directly on the spine. Move along the trapezius and down the left hand side of the spine. 'Jump' over the spine and up the right side and over to the right shoulder. Move back down the right side jumping the spine again and continue up the left side and back along the trapezius. Repeat.

Cupped Hands Percussion

Cup your hands and follow the same route as praying hands, lightly cupping the back. Zigzag between the shoulder blades down and back up. Bend down behind the client. Cup your hand and gently rest your elbow on the sacrum. Use your elbow as a lever, slowly but firmly pat between the shoulder blades. This stimulates the lungs.

Grounding

With thumb and forefinger, apply pressure on either side of the Achilles tendon on the bladder and kidney points. This will help ground the client. Walk round to the front and wait for them to open their eyes.

Additional techniques to integrate with the sequence

The following techniques can all be carried out with the client sitting in the chair. While the basic 20-minute sequence is profoundly effective as a stand-alone treatment, practitioners who have skills in other therapies will discover that they can integrate aspects of other therapeutic treatments to enhance the sequence. We have given you a few of our favourite extra techniques that will add considerable therapeutic value to your sessions. Common sense and experience will guide you as to where they can be included in the sequence but we have indicated where to integrate some of them.

Whole Body Analysis

If you are giving a longer session and the client has specific problems, take note of areas of tension – and take time to make a quick assessment of the client, which will form a basis for attention to any problem areas.

Observe alignment of the whole body. Is one shoulder or ear higher than the other? Is one side of the pelvis higher than the other or rotated forward? Check how the client stands. Is one foot further forward? Is the head turned more to the left or right than facing straight ahead? Are there any curvatures on the spine? Are there areas of hypertonicity on the back muscles? If uneven shoulders straighten out when the client sits down, then the problem will originate from the lower back.

Warm-up

Zigzag Finger Spread

This technique is particularly beneficial on sensitive areas or as a gentle and soothing introduction to your touch. It allows initial contact to the sensitive area, where direct pressure may be uncomfortable. Start at the top left shoulder and work in zigzag lines, traversing down and up again across the back. Keep contact with just the pads of the fingers, thumb and outer edge of the hand. As you move away, spread your fingers and bring them back together as you draw your hand back. If you can co-ordinate well, use both hands.

Single Palm Press

Use this technique at any time during the sequence to loosen tight back muscles. Move to the left side of the client, and with the heel of your right hand, fingers pointing outwards, move the muscles away from the spine from the trapezius to the sacrum – repeat on the other side. This should be a rhythmical rocking motion, using your body weight to lean.

Spinal Circles

With your thumbs, work down the spine in a circular motion away from the spine – from T1 to the base of the sacrum. These circles may be right against the vertebrae and considerable time may be taken over this technique. Use any time in the sequence, but it is particularly useful before working on the nine points with elbow pressure when the client has spasms and trigger points in the erector spinae muscles.

Decompression Move

Using the heels of both hands, work on either side of the spine from the trapezius to the bottom of the thoracic spine. Do not at any time put any direct pressure on the spine. Use an upward intention to the pressure and a gentle jiggle to release the fascia. For maximum release, ask the client to take a deep breath and as they breathe out, apply pressure at intervals all the way down either side of the thoracic spine. This is a powerful move so start gently. You may hear a few clicks as the vertebrae decompress.

Lower Back Stretch

All stretches need to be held for a minimum of eight seconds. Place the heel of your left hand (fingers pointing diagonally downwards) on the right iliac crest of the client and your right hand (fingers pointing upwards) on the left scapula. Ask the client to take a deep breath, and when they breathe out, stretch on the diagonal with your arms crossed. Repeat this on the opposite side.

The lower back stretch can be adapted to stretch the whole left side of the back, using the same technique as the diagonal stretch, keeping arms crossed, but having both hands on the same side of the client's body. This is a good technique to use after the decompression move or when you observe hypertonicity of the muscles on one side of the back. Make sure the muscles are warm before you attempt a stretch.

Place both hands on either side of the sacrum, fingers pointing towards each other and overlapping; push down and hold – this will gently decompress the spine.

Legs

Starting on the left leg, support client's knee with your left hand and give a slight stretch downwards and in. Using the heel of your right hand, apply pressure down the top and sides of the thigh – start gently as this can be a very sensitive area. After warming up, press firmly at intervals towards the knee. Firstly along the stomach meridian and then the gall bladder meridian. If the client has lower back problems, this may be noticeably more sensitive on one side than the other. When the pressures are comfortable, work five equidistant points along the stomach meridian and then gall bladder. Do this twice.

Lower the leg and warm from the knee to the ankle by squeezing the muscles. Work on the stomach meridian, from just below the tuberosity of the tibia in five equidistant points to just in front of the lateral malleolus. Repeat. Five points on the gall bladder meridian, along the peroneal muscles to the calcaneofibular ligament, just below the ankle bone. Repeat. Finish with five points from behind the knee to the Achilles tendon along the bladder meridian. Brush down the leg and squeeze the foot before replacing on rest.

Arms and Hands

Arm Nerve Stretches

This is a good stretch for anyone with symptoms of carpal tunnel syndrome or any other upper limb repetitive strain disorder.

With the arm by the side of the client, turn their hand until you can feel a resistance. Keeping their hand under gentle tension, (get feedback) straighten their fingers and pull down to stretch. Hold for 15 seconds.

LEG MERIDIANS

Spleen, Liver, Kidney, *Stomach, Gall Bladder, Bladder*

Stomach Meridian
Start at hip bone level
with pubic bone, end
on front of ankle joint
1. ST 31
2. Nameless
3. Nameless
4. Nameless
5. ST 35
6. ST 36
7. Nameless
8. ST 40
9. Nameless
10. ST 41

**Gall Bladder
Meridian**
From the top of the
femur to lower edge
of outer ankle bone
GB Points 1-10
1. GB 30
2. Nameless
3. GB 31
4. Nameless
5. Nameless
6. GB 34
7. Nameless
8. Nameless
9. Nameless
10. GB 40

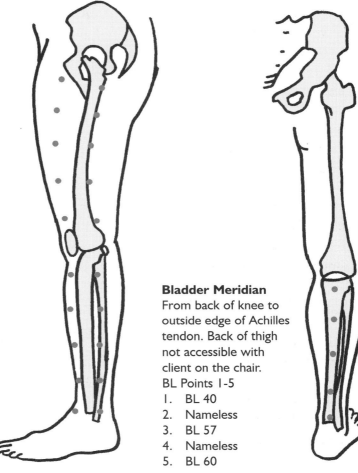

Bladder Meridian
From back of knee to
outside edge of Achilles
tendon. Back of thigh
not accessible with
client on the chair.
BL Points 1-5
1. BL 40
2. Nameless
3. BL 57
4. Nameless
5. BL 60

In the leg work, the Stomach, Gall Bladder and Bladder Meridians are worked on directly, but the Spleen, Liver and Kidney Meridians receive some general stimulation from squeezing and warming up the leg muscles.

Wrist Release

Hold the arm just above the wrist with one hand, and with the other, interlock your fingers with the client's and rotate the wrist firmly, but slowly and gently in both directions using slight traction. Give a pull and shake.

Palm Stretch

Using both hands, interlace your fingers with the client's fingers (whilst their hand is palm up), spreading the palm open. Work on points with thumbs. The stretch is more effective if you cross both of your little fingers over the client's middle finger. The hand and arm work is useful for clients with RSI symptoms. Pay particular attention to the shoulders, the base of the neck and the area around the elbow (H 3, PC 3 and particularly L5). Also point 4 on the triple heater meridian.

Head and Neck

Temple and Ear Massage

During the head massage, use the fingertips and slide them firmly across the forehead. With the tips of your fingers on the temples, move the skin in a circular motion. Massage the ears, starting at the top of the ears to the back pulling towards the back of the head; work all the way to the lobes, using your finger and thumb, squeeze the lobes and give a slight downward pull.

Warming the Occipital Base

After the cupped hand percussion, tip the head forward slightly and with the heel of your hand, rub along the occipital base to warm the area.

Neck Tension and Chronic Problems

Gently tip the head forward and with your fingertips resting on the client's shoulders, work your thumbs up on either side of the cervical spine, from C7 to the occipital base. Be aware of areas of tension and any irregularities in the musculature. If there are, repeat this process whilst slowly moving your thumbs in a circular motion to release any adhesions. You may take your time over this movement.

Continue down the neck and onto the trapezius, circling out towards the shoulder joint, and moving the muscle away from the spine. This will help to remove adhesions around C7 where many people experience stiffness.

Neck Squeeze

Interlace your fingers and turn your palms towards the back of the neck, with your little fingers up against the base of the skull – gently squeeze inwards, working down the trapezius in three movements. Work along either side of the cervical vertebrae with ascending alternate hand movement, taking the muscle between thumb and forefinger.

Pectoral Circles

Start from just below the clavicle (kidney meridian) and working outwards with your fingertips to the space between the pectorals and deltoid (lung meridian). Massage your fingertips in a circular motion all around the anterior rotator cuff muscles.

Chinese Roll

This technique is used extensively in Chinese massage and can be applied to any muscle group anywhere on the body with great effect. Keep the lateral side of the hand in constant contact with the client's muscle. Roll the hand back and forth across the muscle, remaining for several moments on any areas of tension and tightness or at trigger points and acupressure points. This technique is particularly good for working the area where the shoulder and neck meet and also around the rotator cuff muscles.

Shoulder Roll and Shake

Gently grasp lifting and squeezing along the top of the trapezius gradually increasing the pressure and introducing a gentle shake. Grasp the upper trapezius muscles between the heel of the hand and thumb and roll the muscles up and over the top of the shoulder. People with well-developed shoulder muscles appreciate this move.

Scapula Rub

Support the front of the right shoulder with your left hand and with the heel of your right hand rub the scapula in a circular motion, to release any final soreness or tension. Repeat on the other side. This can be included before the final percussion work.

Fascia Release Palm Circles

With the palms of your hands on the base of the spine, gently but firmly move your hands in large circles, first clockwise, then anti-clockwise – this pulls the fascia and releases adhesions from the spine. Work up the length of the spine.

Monkey Circles

Another technique to give your thumbs a break. Curl your fingers and with the back of the fingers between the top two phalangeal joints, knead around the muscles in small circles. Good to use around the neck and for loosening adhesions and trigger points on the sternocleidomastoid muscle.

Tibetan Massage

Make fists, stand behind the client and with straight arms knead firmly down and up and down the erector spinae muscles on either side of the spine.

Soft Tissue Trigger Point and Positional Release Techniques

There are well-documented connections between myofascial trigger point activity and a wide range of whole body dysfunctions. Trigger points appear in muscles stressed from postural imbalances and other traumas both physical and psychological. There are several classic positions for trigger point activity in the muscles of the shoulders and neck and they are commonly found in fibrotic tissue, feeling like a hard pea-sized lump under the fingers. The trigger point itself will be painful when palpated, but will also have a target area to which pain or other symptoms are referred. There are several methods of releasing trigger points, but it is important to bring the muscle back to its normal resting length or else the trigger point will come back. Always warm the muscles first before attempting trigger point release. Apply pressure directly onto the trigger point by direct downward pressure with the thumb or compress the trigger point between thumb and forefinger. In many cases, moving an associated joint to a position where the muscle is at ease and the discomfort is reduced (positional release) will enhance the effect of trigger point release. When the pain disappears, usually after 15 - 30 seconds, the muscle should be stretched passively to its new length. Another method is for the client to introduce an isometric contraction to the muscle whilst the trigger point is compressed by the therapist for at least 15 seconds.

Shoulder Rotations

With the arm fully extended, support and isolate the shoulder joint by placing one hand firmly on the upper trapezius. Rotate the shoulder joint passively in increasingly wider circles in both directions. If the client feels discomfort at any point as the joint is taken through its range of motion, stop and release the area of tension with any of the techniques described above that are appropriate for the area. Normally the monkey circles, Chinese roll or the cross fibre vibration, are the best techniques to use. At the same time, ask the client to visualise that their shoulder is rotating in both directions. Rotate the shoulder joint as before and you will probably find that the discomfort has gone or lessened and that the joint moves more freely.

Sacrum Paddle

In addition to the lower back point work and stretches, you can release the lower back further. Stand directly behind the client, tuck your elbows into your waist and using the heels of both hands gently paddle the sacrum and along the iliac crest with downward pushes using alternate hands.

Neck Release

This technique can be taught to all your clients who experience stiffness when moving the neck through its range of motion. Ask the client to bend the neck to one side as far as they can go without discomfort. Ask them to tap firmly along the length of the extended sternocleidomastoid muscle with the tips of their fingers. Repeat on the other side of the neck. With head bent forward and back of neck muscles extended, ask them to tap the muscles on either side of the spine from the top of the shoulders, up the neck and halfway up the back of the head. This stimulates the underused muscle fibres to prepare for action. Looking straight ahead, 'draw' small circles in both directions with the nose. Turn the head to the left and draw small circles with the chin in both directions, repeat on the other side. This isolates and releases the specific muscles that turn and bend the neck. If practised daily, the neck should remain free from stiffness and discomfort.

Bone Balancing

If you observe that your client's face is out of alignment, probably one eyebrow or one ear higher than the other, this could be the starting point of whole body musculoskeletal dysfunction which in turn can affect hearing, vision, or lead to joint stiffness and circulation problems. Frequently, the mastoid bones are found to be out of balance, which affects the flow of energy elsewhere in the head and throughout the whole body. Stand behind the client and place one forefinger underneath the mastoid bone that is lower, and above the mastoid bone that is higher. Do not press or massage. Just hold the position and try to tune into the subtle change in bone position and energy flow beneath your fingers. Your client may be aware of a shift in the energy flow in their head. If you have the time, you can continue this subtle but very effective bone balancing technique on other parts of the head and face where you can see misalignments.

Releasing C1

C1 or the atlas is the first cervical vertebrae and supports the head and together with C2 the axis, forms a pivot joint that allows the head to move from side to side and up and down. C1 lacks spinal processes and cannot be released the same way as C2 - C7. To check if C1 needs releasing, sit the client up, stand behind them and gently feel into the space below the mastoid process and the maxilla mandibular joint. It should be possible to push the fingers well into the spaces. If one or both sides seem blocked, start vibrating the middle fingers in the spaces as the client turns the head slowly from side to side. Direct the fingers upwards or downwards depending on where the blockage is. After two or three head rotations, you should have created more space behind the ears, indicating that you have successfully released C1. The client may find it easier to turn their head from side to side.

Grounding

At the end of the sequence, to bring the energy down and ground the client, apply thumb pressure to the point in the middle of the palm of the hand on the heart governor meridian on each side simultaneously and gently pull the fingers downwards. Then press the flesh part on either side of the ankle half way between the Achilles tendon and ankle bone on the kidney meridian.

Take the front feet firmly, squeeze and give a downward pull. If the client has removed the shoes, press the solar plexus point in the middle just below the ball of the foot.

The teaching and courses may differ at other colleges, but here is a flavour of the course we run, to illustrate what is involved in becoming a seated acupressure massage practitioner.

The following pictures illustrate some of the 20-minute basic sequence or Kata. It is important to remember that although the work stimulates the flow of energy in the 12 major meridians, not all the points worked are tsubos or acupressure points. The Kata is a rhythmical sequence of moves designed to balance the flow of energy to all parts of the body and throughout the session, many acupressure points are directly stimulated with thumb and elbow pressures.

The Chair

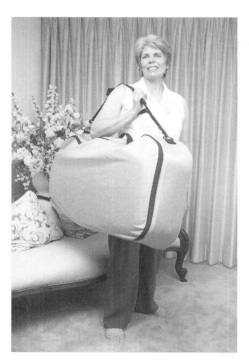

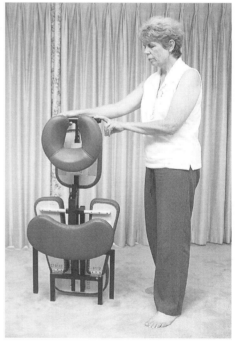

Most chairs come with a carry case. This not only makes the chair totally portable, keeps the chair clean and is more hygienic, but ensures that the chair stays looking good for longer, particularly if your work entails client visits.

Remove the chair from the case and stand it upright.

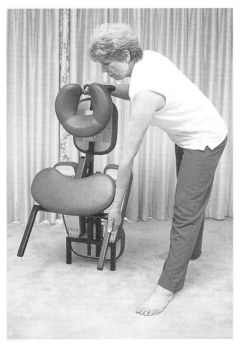

Move the 'A' frame out on the chair.

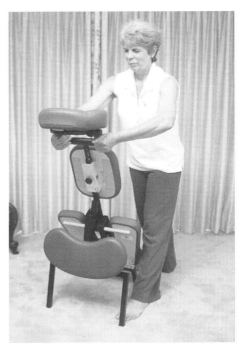

Pressing the knobs on either side of the crossbar, just above the chest piece, will allow you to raise and adjust the headrest.

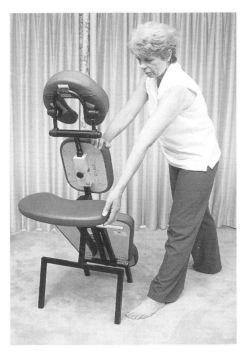

There are three positions for the armrest. Select the position most suitable for you and your client.

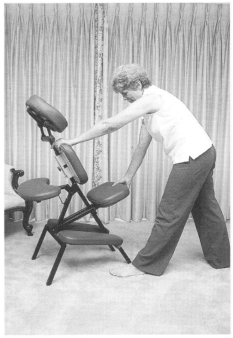

Raise the seat to the correct height for you and your client and ensure that it is secure.

Double Palm Press

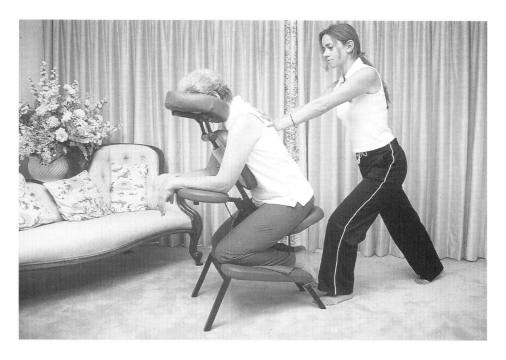

It is important to keep both arms straight as this helps the energy to flow freely and enables the practitioner to let their body weight sink through their arms. Keep the back leg straight to allow the pressure to be applied at 90 degrees to the client's back. Remember to shuffle back with the back foot as you move down the back. This helps to keep your back straight as you work.

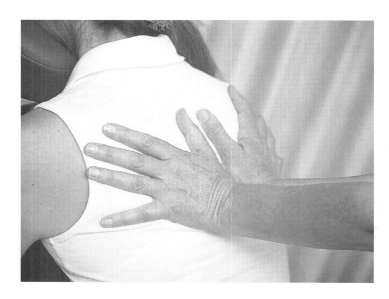

Place your hands on either side of the spine, thumbs pointing upwards. Start level with the scapula.

Archer Press

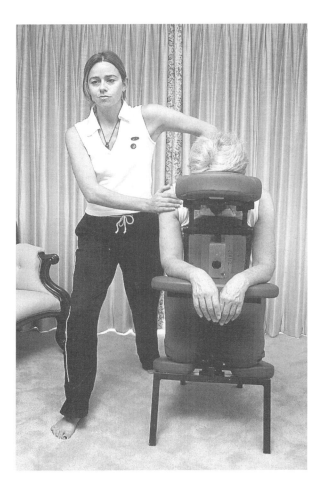

Imagine moving into your front knee, keeping your shoulders square and looking straight ahead.

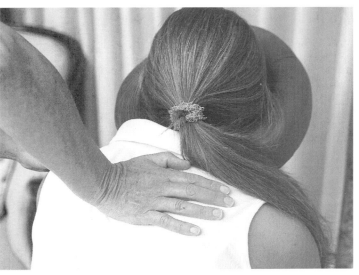

Keep your elbow up and ensure that your fingers are pointing away from you. Allow the pressure to be applied through the heel of your hand and move away from the spine and towards the client's scapula.

Forearm Press

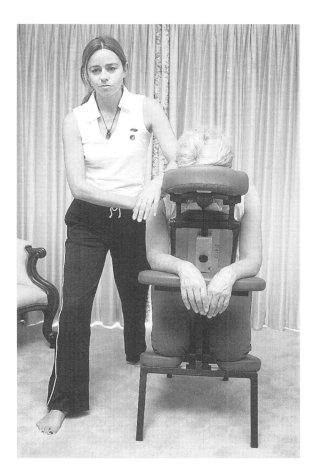

It is easier to get above the client and sink down into the top of the trapezius, rather than trying to use your strength. Ensure that you angle your arm slightly, turning your palm away from you to use the fleshy part of your forearm. Sink in for three points, moving along the trapezius, starting as close to the neck/shoulder junction as possible and ending just in front of the acromion process. Just work on the muscle and not the bone.

Nine Points

Small Intestine SI 14 and Bladder Meridians BL 11-18

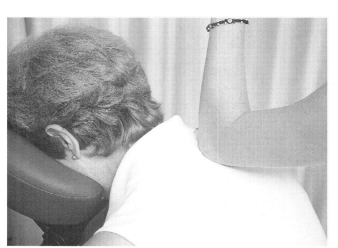

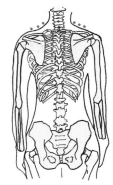

The first of the nine points is located between C7 and T1 in the trapezius and is SI 14.

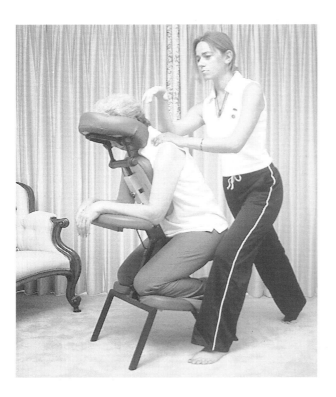

Keep your hands soft and direct the pressure at 90 degrees to the client's back. Allow your weight to sink in slightly, by flexing your front knee. Always go more gently on the first line of points to assess the pressure. It is important at this point to check that the client is comfortable with the pressure. It is quite a common mistake for practitioners to work too far away from the spine. This will lead to discomfort as the pressure is then applied to the head of the ribs. Make sure that you are close to the spine along the erector spinae muscles, but not actually on the spine.

Make sure that you lift the pressure off as you shuffle back with your back leg, move down the erector spinae muscle, one vertebrae at a time to point 9. Points 2 - 9 are on the bladder meridian.

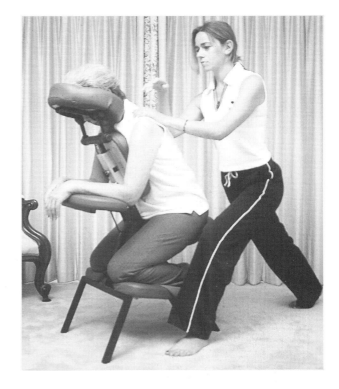

Four Scapula Points

Small Intestine SI 13 and Bladder Meridian Bl. 37,39,41

These points are on the medial border of the scapula starting in line with the superior angle of the scapula and moving downwards in a straight line ending in line with the inferior angle of the scapula. They are equidistant and fairly close to the nine points. Point 1 is SI 13, points 2, 3 and 4 are on the bladder meridian. The bladder meridian is the longest meridian in the body starting at the inside corner of the eye and ending on BL 67 on the outer edge of the little toe by the nail bed.

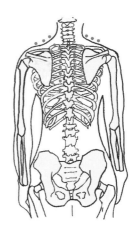

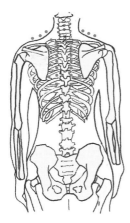

Trapezius Crest Points

Gall Bladder Meridian GB21 and Large Intestine Meridian Ll16

Make sure you start very close into the neck and try to get above the points to allow your weight to sink in. Point 2 is GB 21, midway between the interspinous space C7-TH1 and the tip of the acromion on the trapezius muscle at its highest point on the shoulder. Point 3 LI 16 is in the depression behind the acromioclavicular articulation.

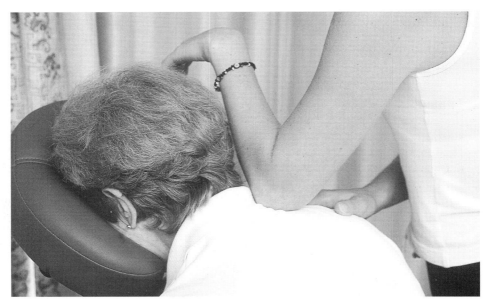

Arm Squeeze

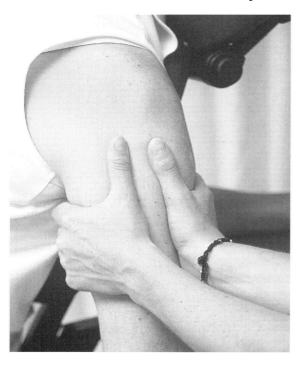

*Squeeze the whole
length of the arm in
five positions, starting
at the deltoid muscle
and ending at the wrist.*

Deltoid To Elbow

Large Intestine Meridian LI 14,

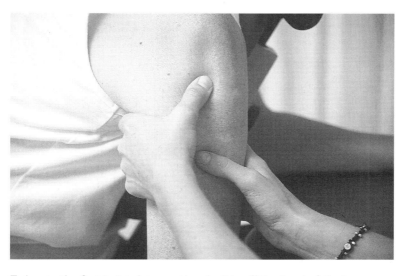

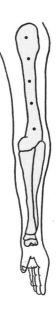

*To locate the first point, let your thumb slide off the head of the humerus
and approximately two inches down into the deltoid. 'Walk' down 5
points in a hand over hand motion to the 5th point just above the elbow
crease on the lateral border of the triceps muscle.*

Posterior Forearm
Large Intestine Meridian LI 11,9,7,5

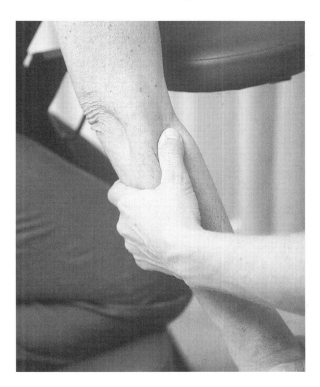

Turn the hand so that the client's thumb is facing you. Start immediately below the elbow crease in the brachioradialis muscle. This point, LI 11 can often be tender, particularly if the client has tennis elbow or RSI type symptoms. Apply pressure to 5 points ending at LI 5.

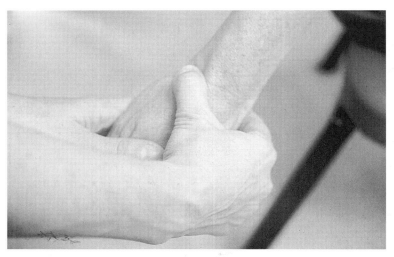

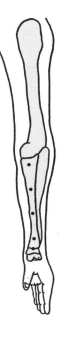

Point 5, LI 5 is located midway between the tendons of the extensor pollicis brevis and longus muscles of the wrist. If you are working on the left arm, use your right thumb to apply pressure.

Triple Heater Meridian

(Also known as Triple Warmer or Sanjiao Channel) TH 9, 5, 4

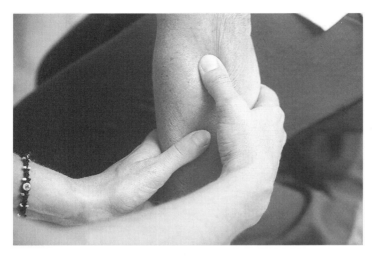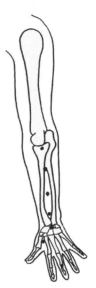

With the back of the client's hand facing you, start just below the elbow and 'walk down' between the radius and ulna, in a hand over hand motion for 5 points to the wrist. Point 5 TH 4 lies in the depression between the tendons of the extensor muscles in the transverse crease of the wrist, in the middle of the wrist joint.

Small Intestine Meridian

SI 8, 7, 6, 5

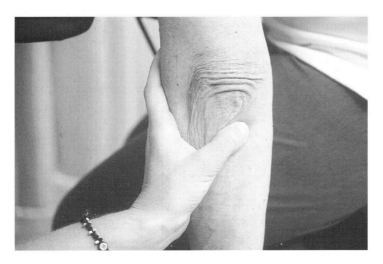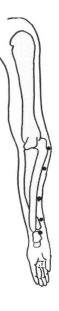

With the little finger facing you, press SI 8 starting just below the elbow in the groove under the medial epicondyle, work 5 points behind the ulna down to the wrist.

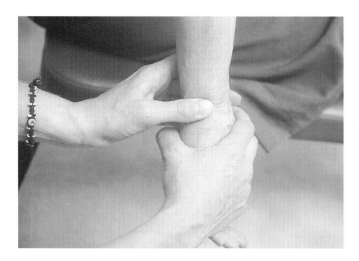

The fifth small intestine point at the side of the wrist. SI 5 lies in the depression between the styloid process and pisiform bone at the little finger side of the wrist.

Hands

Hand Spread

Using the heel of your hands and thumbs, spread the back of the hand.

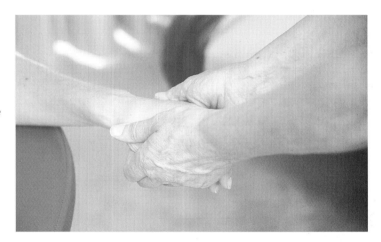

Thumb Strokes

With your fingers supporting the underside of the client's hand, use your thumbs to stroke down between the outer metacarpals.

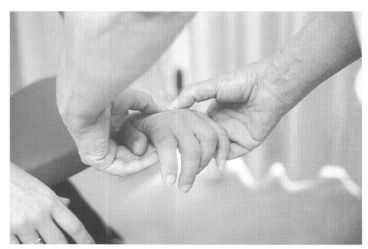

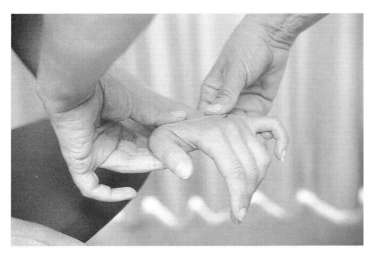

Turn your wrists so your thumbs are facing you as a continuous movement.

Stroke down to the webbing.

Heart Meridian
H. 3, 4, 7

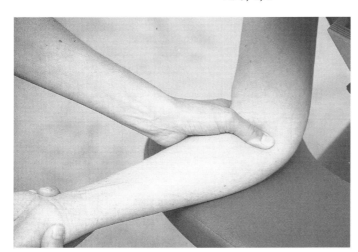

Start just below the elbow crease. H.3 on the anterior forearm and work five points to the wrist points 4 and 5 are H.4 and H.7

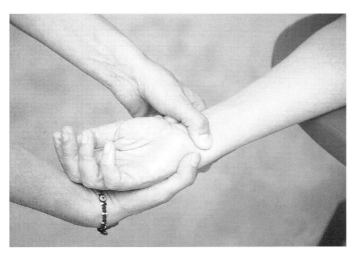

Point 5, H.7 is located on the palmar side of the wrist.

Heart Protector Meridian

HP 3, 4, 6, 7

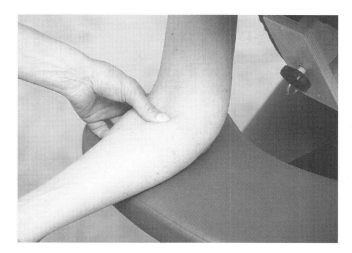

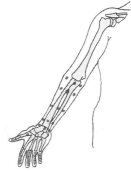

Point 1 is located just below the elbow crease in the middle of the anterior forearm.

Palm Spread

Using the heels of your hands and thumbs, spread the palm of the hand. This feels great, particularly if the client operates machinery or uses the keyboard for much of the time.

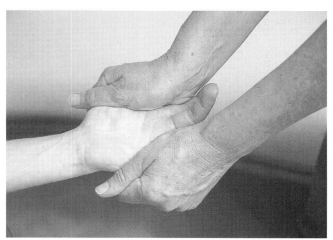

Thumb Strokes

Stroke down between the outer metacarpals twice and then mobilise twice.

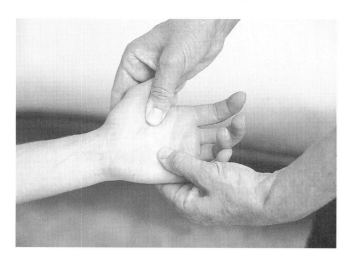

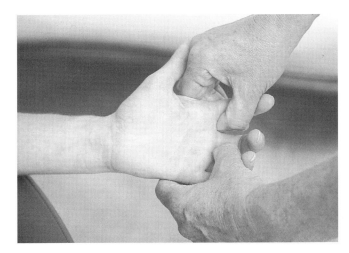

Finish by bringing your fingers through the webbing

Lung 10

Apply pressure with your thumb in the middle of the first metacarpal bone to the centre of thenar eminence.
(not shown)

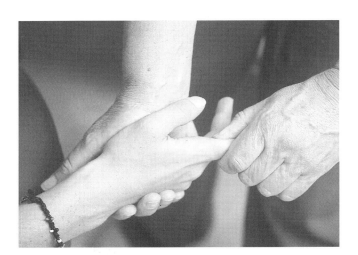

Coin Rubs

Using your thumb and forefinger, rub the top and bottom of the thumb from the base to the tip and then rub down the sides. Repeat for each finger.

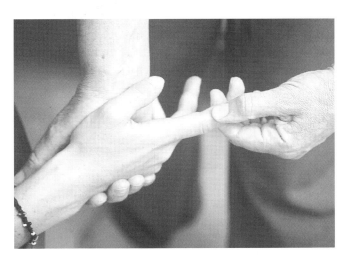

Squeeze either side of the nail. Six meridians end or start at the fingers. Yin meridians, Lung, Heart Protector and Heart end on the fingers. Yang meridians, Large Intestine, Triple Heater and Small Intestine start on the fingers.

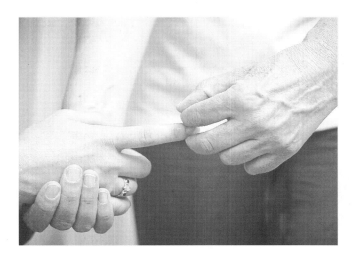

Finger Flicks

Sandwich the tip of the finger between the first phalangeal joints of the index and middle finger. Press the tip of the thumb against the index finger to stabilise and pull off. You should hear a satisfying 'click'. Make sure you direct the energy away from your own body.

Arm Stretch

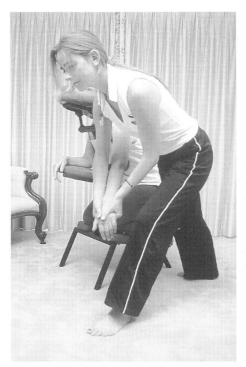

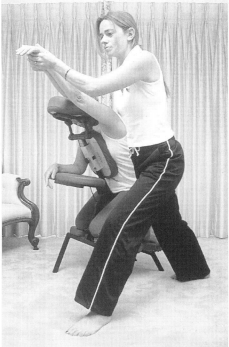

Take the arm from the arm rest and give it a gentle downwards pull. Hold either side of the hand and keep it under tension as you raise the arm. Tell the client to take a deep breath

On the client's out breath, raise clients arm up and slightly away from their body. This will stretch the infraspinatus, teres minor and supraspinatus muscles. Hold the stretch for a few seconds and gently vibrate the arm. Your body should be in lunge position with your front knee bent.

Lower Back
Bladder Meridian Bl 19-28 and BL 48, 29, 34, 35

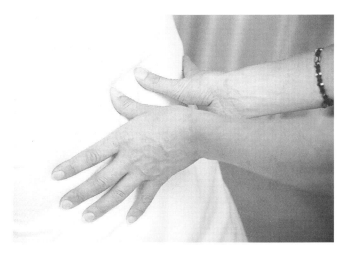

The first point is located on either side of the spine in the erector spinae muscle, just between thoracic vertebrae 9 and 10. Move down between each vertebra for 9 points. The last point should end between Lumbar 5 and Sacrum 1.

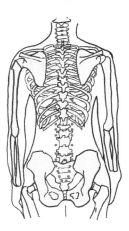

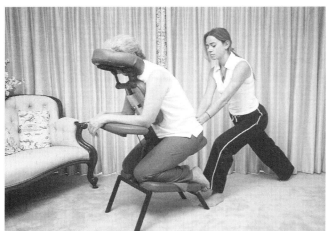

As you move down the lower back with thumb pressures, your stance will widen. Always keep the back leg straight.

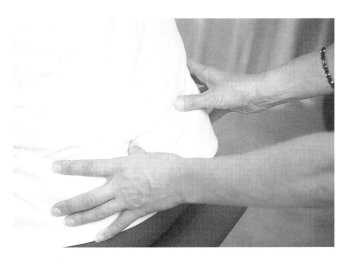

The first sacrum point is located at the top of the sacrum near the outer edges. Follow the shape of the sacrum in for points 2, 3, and 4 on the posterior sacral foramina.

The 4th point, Bl 35 is located above the coccyx on either side of the sacral vertebrae.

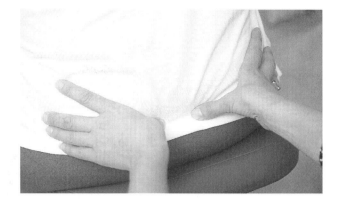

Neck Lines *(3 lines, 5 points)*
Governing Vessel GV 15 and Gall Bladder GB 20,12

Starting close to the cervical spine level with C3, use the pad of the thumb to move the muscle away from the spine. Gently rest your fingers on the other side of the neck and be careful not to dig the thumb in. Continue down for 5 points, repeating each line twice. Move further away from the spine by one thumb width, for the start of each new line.

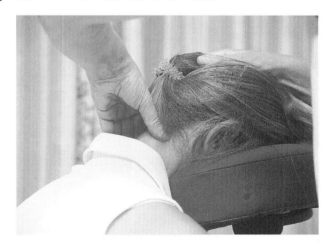

Trapezius Crest Points
Small Intestine SI 15

Stand facing the back of the client and starting laterally, move in along the trapezius crest for 3 points (point 1 shown)

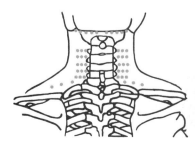

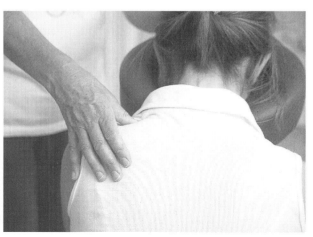

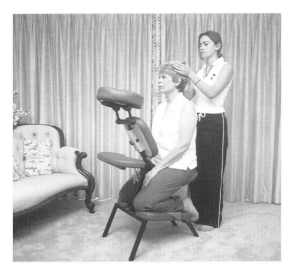

Sit The Client Up

When you sit the client up, centre them and gently raise the head by placing your palms above their ears and lifting slightly.

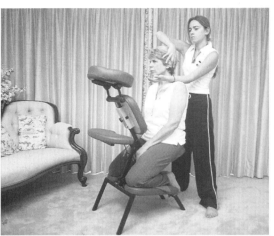

Neck Stretch

Stretch the left side of the neck first, and as shown place your right forearm, palm facing upwards on the client's right shoulder. Bring your left arm around so your fingers are holding on either side of the right ear.

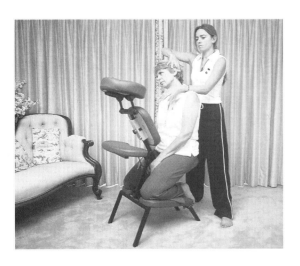

Ask the client to take a deep breath, and as they exhale, pronate your right forearm and press down on the trapezius. With your forearm, gently stretch upwards and move the neck to the left. You should be using about seventy per cent downward pressure and thirty per cent across. It is important not to let your elbow rest on the client's head as you are stretching the neck over. Hold the stretch for a few seconds and release slowly.

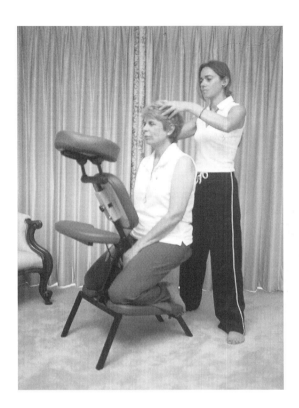

Scalp Massage

Using the pads of your fingers, firmly move them over the scalp in a circular motion. The scalp should move under your fingers. This is followed by scalp lifts.

Cupped Hands Percussion

Starting near the base of the skull, work upwards, just left of the centerline, to the front of the hairline on the frontal bone. Work all around the crown in a full circle to the front again. Finish by working downwards, just right of the centerline. Make sure you have a cushion effect with your hands together creating a pocket of air and keep your wrists soft. This move stimulates the gall bladder meridian.

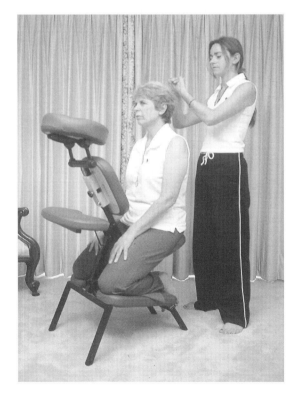

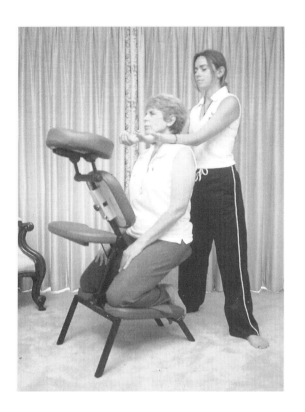

Double Forearm Press

Using your forearms, start with palm facing upwards, resting on the trapezius. Stand with your toes pointing outwards and ask the client to take a deep breath.

As the client exhales, flex your knees and apply pressure in three positions along the trapezius as you pronate your forearms.

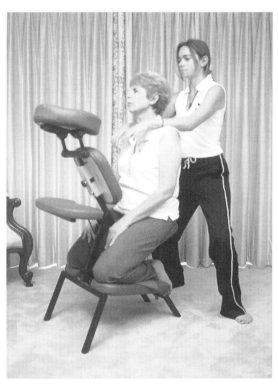

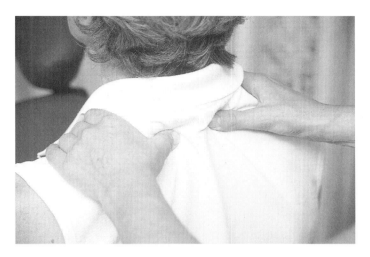

Thumb Squeeze Rotations

Starting on either side of the 1st thoracic vertebrae, move your thumbs in a circular motion outward along the trapezius.

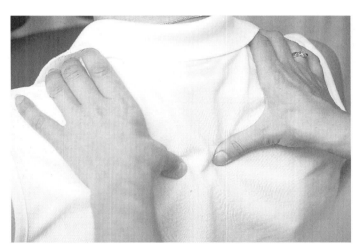

Then work down on either side of the thoracic vertebrae with your fingers still gently resting on the top of the shoulders.

Shoulder Squeeze

Squeeze the top of the trapezius in three positions, moving outwards towards the deltoid. Lift the muscle as you do this, taking care not to pinch. Then squeeze down the upper arm along the deltoid, lifting the muscle away from the bone.

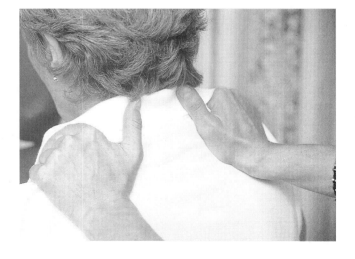

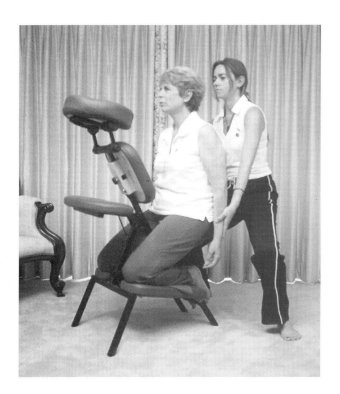

Chicken Wing Stretch

Slide your hands down the client's arm and take the back of their forearm so the palms of their hands are facing forwards.

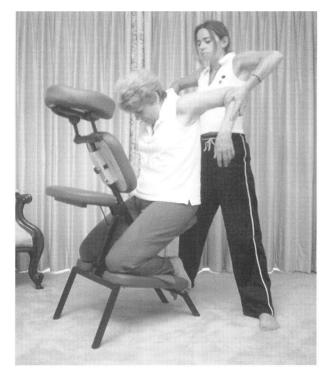

Ask the client to take a deep breath, and as they exhale, drop their head forward. As the client breathes out, raise their arms behind them, keeping their elbows pointing out at 45 degrees. Ask them to tell you when they can feel a good stretch and hold for 8 seconds.

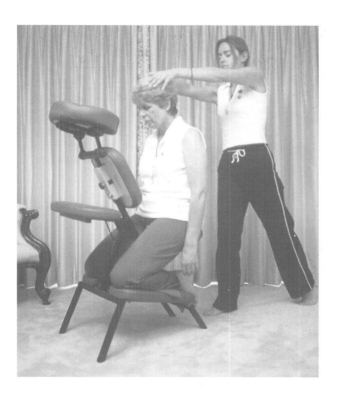

Full and Final Brush Down

Place your hands on the client's head and let the energy gather for a moment.

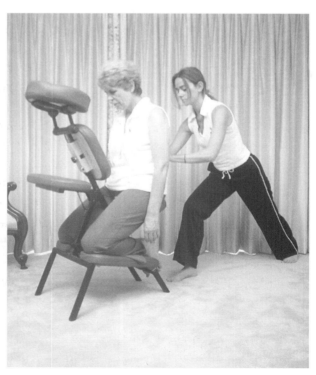

Sweep briskly down the back, repeat two more times and then once down the arms.

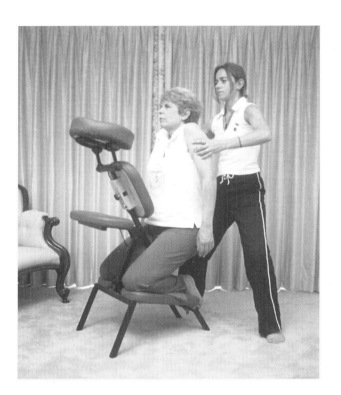

Shoulder Lifts

Take the arms at the deltoid, taking care not to pinch. Say to the client, "Take a deep breath and when I drop your shoulders, let your breath go".

Lift the client's shoulders and briskly 'throw' down their arms. Repeat this. On the third time, lift their arms, but just let them drop ready to go straight into the hacking.

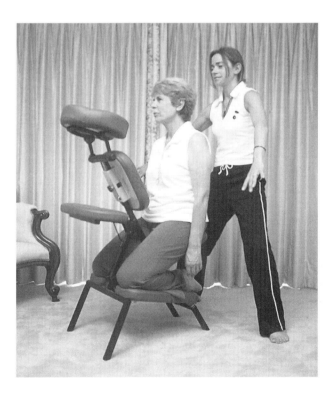

Percussion

The following percussion moves should only be carried out over soft tissue and not directly on the bone.

Hacking

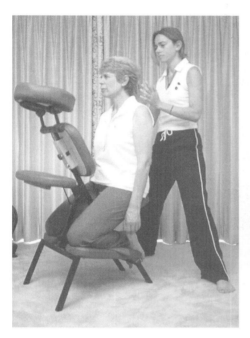

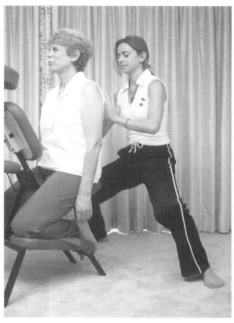

Start the hacking with one hand on either side of the shoulder. Your fingers should be open and wrists loose. Start close into the neck and move out across the top of the trapezius and back in again.

Hack down either side of the spine and back up again and repeat.

Praying Hands

Press your hands together and move your elbows out to 90 degrees, keeping your fingers open and your wrists loose. Start on the left shoulder and move out along the top of the trapezius and back in before going down the left of the spine, 'jump' over the spine and back up the right. Follow the same route as for the hacking.

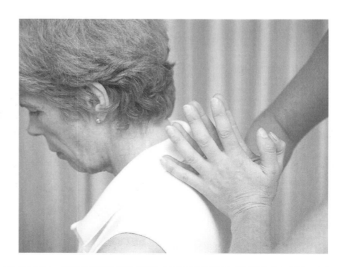

Cupped Hands

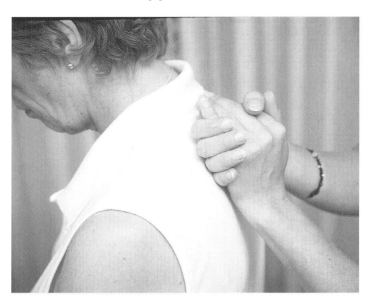

Place one hand over the other as if you are holding a small ball. Try to keep your hands air tight as this will offer a cushioning effect to the client. As with all the percussion moves, keep your wrists loose and follow the same route as before. End the cupped hands with stitching, i.e. zigzagging from one side of the back to the other. This integrates both sides of the back.

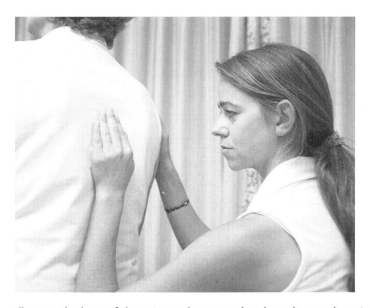

Place your elbow at the base of the spine and cup your hand gently over the spine, making a "channel" with your third finger and heel of your hand, so there is no direct pressure on the spine. Keeping your wrist soft, cup your hand a few times over the solar plexus area of the back.

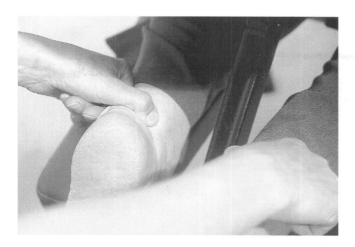

Ground the client by applying pressure gently to either side of the Achilles tendon. Your thumbs should be facing each other. This is on the kidney meridian.

Legs

Stomach and Gall Bladder and Bladder Meridians ST 31-41, GB 29-40, Bl 55-60

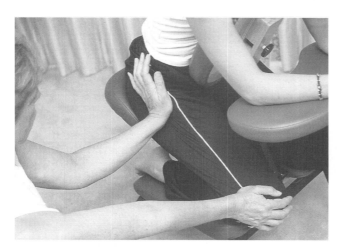

Begin by gently applying pressure to just above the knee to stretch the quadriceps femoris. With the heel of the other hand, work in intervals down the top of the thigh (stomach meridian), and side of the thigh (gall bladder meridian as shown). Start gently as these points are often very sensitive and you may need to do this two or three times until the muscles relax.

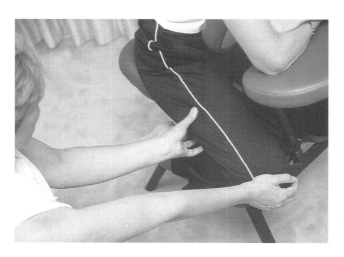

Using thumb pressure, work in equidistant points along the two meridians. Line 1, stomach meridian, with point 1 in the iliacus and ending at the base of the rectus femoris, just above the patella. Line 2, gall bladder meridian working from the hip joint, along the vastus lateralis, ending just above the knee.

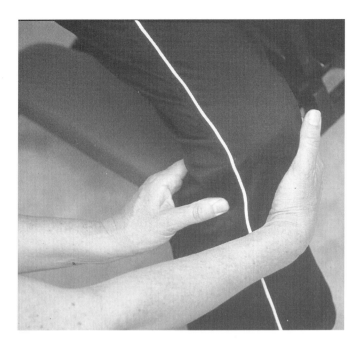

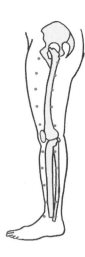

Supporting the inside of the knee, apply pressure on the second line – gall bladder, starting just below the head of the fibula. The next 4 points are equidistant. (Point 5 shown in top diagram).

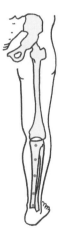

Additional Techniques

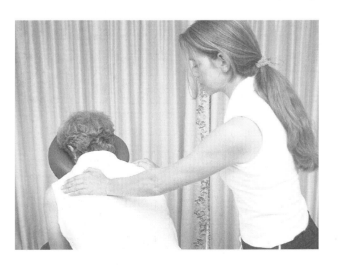

Single Palm Press

Stand behind the client, just to one side and using the heel of the hand with your fingers pointing away from the spine, lean your body weight in and move the heel of your hand towards your fingers, easing the muscles away from the spine.

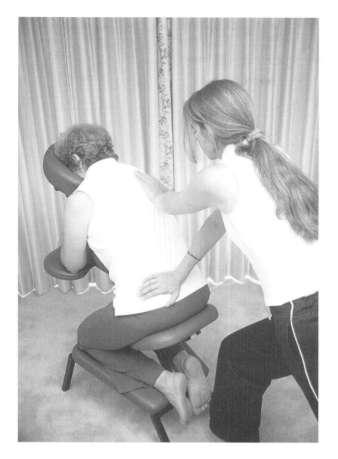

Lower Back Stretch

Stand with a wide stance, so you are able to sink your body weight into this stretch. Crossing hands over each other, place one hand around the scapula, and the other around the sacrum. Ask the client to take a deep breath and as they breathe out, flex your front knee and move your hands away from each other to give a good stretch. Hold for a minimum of 8 seconds.

Repeat the stretch for both sides as well as on the diagonal. You may need to alter your stance to get the most effective lean.

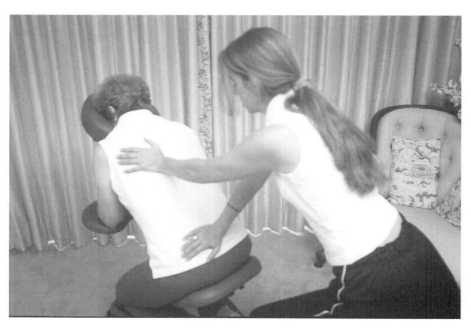

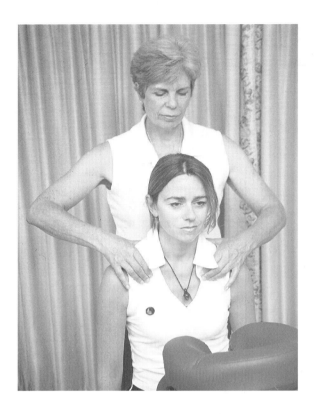

Pectoral Circles
Lung, Liver and Stomach Meridians

Starting above the clavicle, move outwards along the sternocleidomastoid and trapezius in a circular motion, being careful to use only the pads of your fingers. Move to just below the clavicle and using the pads of your fingers again in a circular motion work along the pectoralis major.

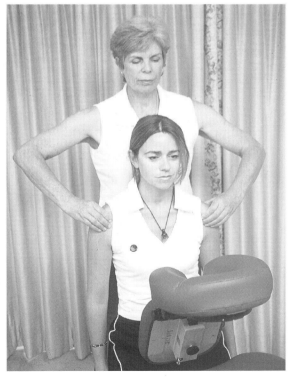

Continue outwards to the acromioclavicular articulation where a great deal of stiffness is often found. This move is addressing the lung, liver and stomach meridians.

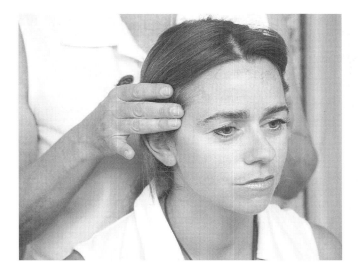

Temple Massage

This area will often be the focus of much tension. It is extremely important that no pressure is used on the area. Using the pads of the fingers, work in a circular motion, moving the fascia around and forwards to release tension around the sphenoid bone – this can help with sinus problems, headaches and migraines.

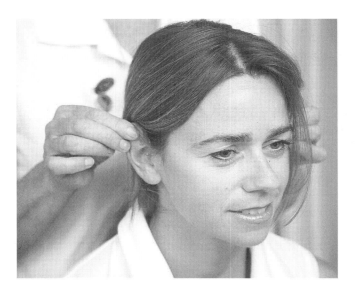

Ear Work

Ears are often sensitive and hold tension. There are numerous acupuncture points on the ear – with some therapies dedicated entirely to this practice. The ears also relate to the nervous, circulatory and digestive systems. By working along the outer edge of the ear, around to the lower lobe, areas of tension may be located and massaged by moving your forefinger outwards to the outer edge.

Additional Hand And Arm Work

These techniques are helpful in the treatment of Repetitive Strain Injury, Carpal Tunnel Syndrome and for people spending large amounts of time on a keyboard.

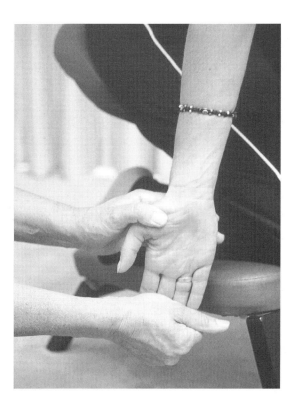

Arm Nerve Stretch

With the arm by the side of the client, turn their hand until you can feel a resistance. Keeping their hand under gentle tension, (get feedback) straighten their fingers and pull down to stretch. Hold for 15 seconds.

Palm Stretch

Interlace your fingers with the client's hand, with your little fingers crossing over each other at the client's middle finger. Using your thumbs, start from the middle of the hand and stroke outwards spreading the palm. This will give a stronger stretch than the palm spread and is particularly good for computer operators etc.

Wrist Release

Firmly supporting the underside of the wrist with one hand, interlace the fingers of the other hand with the client's hand. Gently mobilise the wrist and work in a circular motion in both directions. Flex and extend the wrist and offer gentle traction.

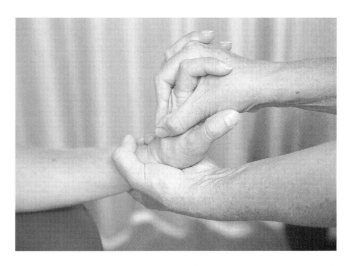

Arm Nerve Stretch

Extend arm fully, shoulder height, turn palm 90 degrees to wrist and 'push' against an imaginary wall.

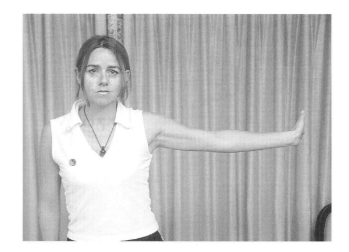

If you need to increase the stretch, lean your head away from the arm being stretched. Remember to always stay within your comfort zone for any stretches.

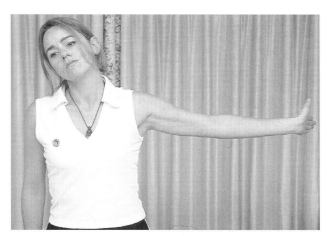

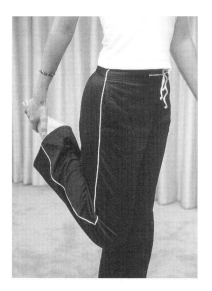

Quadriceps Stretch

For optimum results these stretches should be held for one minute and repeated twice on each side.

Lumbar Stretch

For optimum results, these stretches should be held for one minute and repeated twice on each side.

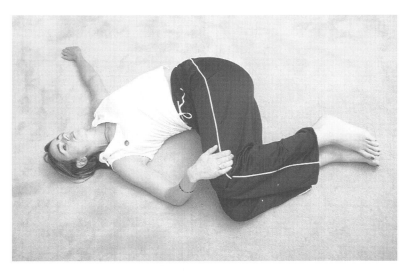

Lie on your back and bring your knees up to your chest at right angles. Keep your hands flat on the floor, palms down at 90 degrees to your body. Exhale and let your knees drop over to one side, whilst keeping your opposite shoulder on the floor. Stay within your comfort zone and do not stretch to the maximum limit.

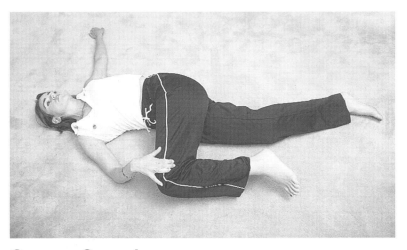

Sacrum Stretch

Lie on your back with your arms on the floor, palms down at 90 degrees to your body. Raise the left leg and bend to a right angle; use your right hand on your left knee to bring it round to the right side. Start with a gentle stretch and don't worry if you can't reach the floor on the other side.

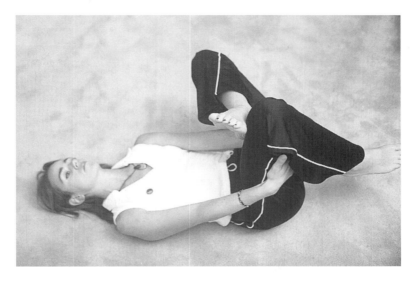

Gluteal Stretch

Lie on the floor and bend your right knee up to your chest. Cross your left foot over onto your right leg and link your hands under your right knee. Let your left knee drop out and gently increase the stretch by pulling on your arms. This will stretch the left gluteal muscle. Make sure when you are doing this stretch that your neck is relaxed and use a pillow if necessary.

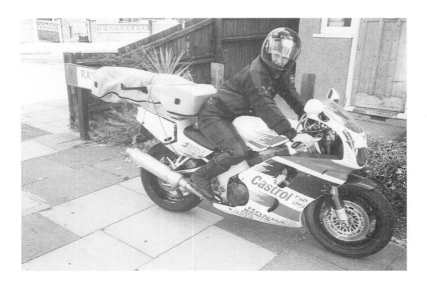

Have bike, have chair, no problem. One of our more adventurous students coming to a practise session on her motorbike.

ACUPRESSURE MASSAGE CASE STUDIES

The training courses in seated acupressure massage are for practitioners with a minimum of a recognized qualification in Anatomy, Physiology and massage. Students are required to present case studies as part of their assessment and as practice makes perfect, at this school, we ask for a minimum of 75 documented practice sessions. The course is in two parts with 4 - 6 weeks between and students are expected to have done 20 - 30 practise sessions before they come back for part 2.

Programme Objectives

1. To provide students with an ongoing record of client treatments.
2. To allow students to develop history taking and interviewing skills.
3. To allow objective assessment of treatment effectiveness.
4. To enable students to integrate their professional knowledge and training.
5. To assist the future development of acupressure knowledge and techniques.
6. To allow for discussion with Tutors on specific areas of concern.

Requirements

Complete and document 75 practice sessions. These are made up of:

- 25 individual sessions – these clients would require screening to ascertain their suitability and a record of name, address, date of massage and any findings; a space should be left for the client's signature and any comments they have.
- 50 case studies, to consist of 5 massage sessions on 10 different clients. If you do not have access to 10 clients, you may massage some of your group 10 times to make up the 50.

All case study volunteers must be fully informed that they are assisting you in your training and that the information taken is made available to the examiner. They may also be contacted to verify the practise sessions.

Documentation

All clients must have an initial completed record form with notes for subsequent visits. These should include the following details:

1. Name, address, telephone number and date of acupressure massage.
2. Medical history and current state of health, diet/lifestyle etc.
3. Physical responses to treatment.
4. Emotional responses during and after treatment.
5. The client's opinion of any progress made.
6. On follow-up appointments, how the client has felt since last the acupressure massage (mental and physical changes).
7. What complaints did the client have at the start of the session – have they been alleviated.
8. You may also want to add occasionally the length of time it took to complete the sequence and if you needed to refer to notes etc.

A numerical rating scheme may be useful to determine sensitive acupressure points:

0	=	No discomfort at all
1	=	Very slight discomfort
2	=	Uncomfortable
3	=	Painful
4	=	Very painful
5	=	Unbearable

This will give the therapist an indication of how the client may be improving over the course of the treatments.

When you have your last session with each client, ask them to write a short note on how they felt they may have benefited from the massages. This does not apply to the individual sessions.

Examination

The exam is for students of seated acupressure massage to be assessed for practitioner level. Successful students will be awarded a certificate of competence, which will enable them to become insured to practice this therapy. Completed case studies must be received at least a week before the exam date. Retain copies for yourself as the originals will be kept on file. Examination is by appointment and will consist of an oral test and

20-minute practical. Students may be asked any information included in the training notes and on subjects discussed during the training.

Chapter 6
Marketing Yourself As A Practitioner

Managing Your Business

Traditionally, practitioners are reluctant to see themselves as business people, and in the early days of building a practice, many of us even feel uncomfortable about asking for our fee at the end of a treatment. That improves with time of course, but practitioners of seated acupressure massage who are planning to secure contracts in the business world, do not have time to be coy about the value of the service they are offering. When approaching a company with your proposal, you need to be professional and confident.

Preparation is the key to success in any business and that means sitting down and writing a business plan and setting up a simple book-keeping system. If you need help with this, in the UK, Barclays Bank and the Nat West have excellent, 'Starting or Running Your Business' packs, or you can contact your local Enterprise Council and local Business Link for help. Both run inexpensive workshops on all aspects of starting and running a business. One of our students also obtained funding from a similar agency in the Midlands that covered the costs of her training, massage chair and advertising costs. The local Inland Revenue Office will give you guidance on your tax returns and National Insurance payments.

If you want to borrow money from the bank to set up your business, you need to present a business plan to them, but even if you are not borrowing money, a business plan will help you to stay focused about your own goals. Before you start to write your business plan, it might help you to think about the following points.

Business Name
Does it give you the right image?

Business/Personal History
What experience do you have for this activity?

Personal Aims and Objectives
What do you want from the business apart from profit?

Aims and Objectives of the Business
Where do you want it to be in a few years time?

In addition, think about key people, market research, advertising and promotion plans, premises and equipment, on-going training, relevant legal matters such as contracts or consumer laws and financial structure, capital, survival income and first three years profit projection. In short, your plan should include:

- Statement of overall business aims. Keep it short and specific.
- Target market e.g. private or business sector.
- Why your product/service is special.
- Resources that you will need.
- What price you will charge and how have you determined it.
- How you will promote your business.
- Set-up costs, fixed monthly costs, cash flow.
- General book-keeping.

You cannot manage your money if you do not know how much you are earning or where it is going, so keeping accurate and up-to-date records and accounts is important. You are required to keep them by law, but they are vital for calculating your tax returns. There is no need for a complicated system, just use common sense. The basics include:

1. A concertina-type file – divide the sections into months and keep all your business-related receipts in the relevant month's partition.

2. An accounts ledger – record all your purchase items for the tax year, month by month in one section. Number your receipts and record the number against the purchase item. Show your income month by month in another section.

3. If you have a computer, make up your own record of expenses and income and keep it updated. Reconcile purchases and payments with your monthly bank statement.

4. You may not be VAT registered to begin with but keep a VAT column going. If your business grows to a point where you have to register, then you can claim VAT for two retrospective years.

Helpful Tips To Promote Yourself Within The Corporate Sector

Target Market

Identify the types of company you are going to contact and formulate a package tailored to their requirements. It may be an area in which you have a particular interest, or an environment where you have previously worked, so that you can personalise it. It is much easier to 'sell' something that you have a better knowledge of.

Collecting Information

Find out as much as you can about the company that you are going to see – either before you visit, or when you begin the meeting. Don't just try to sell your service before finding out what problems the staff and employers are having. What levels of stress are the staff under? Does the company have shift workers? How many employees do they have? What other services do they offer to their employees to reduce stress? What sort of hours do the staff work at the VDU's? Do they have a problem with absenteeism, RSI, back pain etc?

Look Professional

Spend as much as you can afford on your brochure and business cards. Make up a folder with some information to support your presentation. It is a good idea to leave some information on what you do and a scale of fees. It is also beneficial if you can work with someone else, as organisations prefer to deal with other companies, even if it is only someone who covers for you if you are on holiday or sick.

Pricing

When you present your costs, be confident. Remember the service you are offering may end up saving the company money. Make sure you have thought these out carefully so you know what the cost per head is. If the company asks you for something you have not calculated, or you feel like you have been put on the spot and are not good with figures, write down what they require, and tell them you will send them a written quotation when you have calculated it.

Handling Objections

We Have Group Medical Health Insurance

Medical health insurance is a necessity when it comes to giving people peace of mind and immediate medical attention if required – however it does not offer practical stress management and is rather like 'closing the stable door, after the horse has bolted'.

We Offer Telephone Counselling Services/Individual Counselling

Many people are also unaware of their stress levels, so would not consider confronting issues with counsellors, whilst others may feel that it is admitting weakness to do so.

We Have Company Gym Membership

It is known that although this is a valuable service for those that use it, only 10% of individuals within a company take advantage of these services. Not surprisingly, the employees who use the gym are generally those that least need help.

We Offer Stress Management Seminars

Like any seminars or sales training, these are usually very informative and enable people to understand what happens to the body during a stressful event and they are given tools to deal with it. The seminars may also 'kick-start' an individual to make some life changes, some of which may be extremely helpful. Unfortunately, like New Year resolutions, they are often forgotten. They do not however replace the sort of regular one-on-one attention a practitioner would be able to provide within the workplace.

We Have Company Doctors

Although the employee is assured of first-class medical attention, many problems could be prevented or otherwise dealt with immediately, thus eliminating the need for a visit, additional expense and time out of the office.

The subject of stress in the workplace has been discussed elsewhere in this book, but the information here will help practitioners formulate a concise, corporate presentation.

What may be stressful to one person, may not be to another and would depend entirely on how one interprets, consciously or unconsciously a situation or event. This will determine the individuals' reaction and ultimately the effect on their health. The extent of the effect on their health will depend on the support system the individual has and how important the event is perceived to be.

In the ordinary private lives of employees within a company, one may be sure that there are already a number who are experiencing high levels of stress. For example those who are divorced, single parents, or unhappily married. Those contending with bereavement, chronic illness, changes in line of work, additional workload or fear of redundancy. Additional stress will place those people in a high-risk category. Judgments about who is the most likely to be unable to cope with added stress are not easy to make – even for the individual themselves.

Stress is known to be a contributor in ninety per cent of disease and illness. A good stress reduction programme can mean fewer lost days at work. Some of the less well-known aspects of stress are the mental and emotional components. These range from forgetfulness, feeling angry, loss of confidence, lack of concentration, problems in making decisions, irritability, depression, withdrawal, feeling explosive, guilty, hopelessness, panic attacks and anxiety, to list only a few. Seated acupressure massage can help alleviate the symptoms of:

- Anxiety and depression.
- Eyestrain.
- Sinus problems.
- Headaches and migraines.
- Insomnia.
- Backache and sciatica (both recent and old injuries).
- Muscular tension.
- Asthma and breathing difficulties.
- Chronic Fatigue Syndrome.
- Repetitive Strain Injury and Carpal Tunnel Syndrome (including the onset or mild symptoms such as tingling, pins and needles and numbness in hands and fingers).
- Menstrual tension.
- Neck tension and whiplash injuries.
- Skin problems (psoriasis, eczema).
- Hypertension.
- Irritable Bowel Syndrome and digestive problems.

It is not unknown for employees suffering high levels of stress or RSI, to sue their employers. To protect the company from the possibility of litigation, the employer must be seen to be addressing this issue. Effective stress management means having a range of ways to reduce stress. In-house treatment would complement the services companies may already offer to staff.

For part of your presentation, you could summarise the corporate benefits on introducing seated acupressure massage as follows:

- Reduces absenteeism.
- Improves morale.
- Demonstrates commitment of management to staff.
- Practical stress management with immediate results.
- Increases productivity.
- Cost neutral.

Aftercare Advice For Clients

Acupressure massage is a non-invasive therapy, which can help reduce the effects of stress and promote a sense of wellbeing. Regular treatments will have a cumulative effect and provide greater benefit than an individual session.

After the massage, you should feel relaxed but energised and alert. You may experience some mild, short-lived reactions as your body responds to the therapy. You may feel light-headed, your muscles may ache, you might feel hot or cold and you might have an emotional release.

In order to assist your body to eliminate toxins after your massage please follow the general advice given below:

- Relax as much as possible
- Drink plenty of plain water
- Eat a light diet
- Reduce tea, coffee and alcohol

Your practitioner will discuss with you other long-term adjustments you could make to manage stress by simple health promoting measures.

Stretching Exercises For Clients And Practitioners

These exercises can either be done as a complete series, or individually depending on individual requirements. Some will ease tension in specific parts of the body, whilst others will help with general relaxation. Stretching should be relaxing and never be painful.

The busier you are, the more important it is to make time for relaxation and stretching exercises. A number of these exercises can be carried out at work, during breaks and even at your desk! To get the maximum benefit from these exercises, they must be carried out regularly – preferably each day.

Each stretch must be held for at least 15 seconds and repeated twice.

Head And Neck

- Head rotation – keeping your head level, slowly turn it from side to side.
- Slowly drop your head sideways moving your right ear towards your right shoulder and push down with your left shoulder – repeat on the other side.
- Stand with feet shoulder distance apart; look down towards right foot

(hold for 15 seconds), dropping left shoulder. Repeat exercise looking towards left foot.

- Drop the lower jaw and open the mouth wide.

Shoulders

- Shrugging shoulders in a circular movement – forwards then backwards.
- Raise your shoulders high and let them drop heavily, whilst letting your breath go.
- Clasp hands behind head, with elbows back – push your chin back. Hold. From this position look down and push your elbows together at the front.
- Clasp hands and push up towards ceiling, palms up – look down.
- Sit upright in a chair with a firm seat. Raise your arms as high as possible and remaining seated drop forward letting your head and arms hang heavily towards the floor.

Arms And Hands

- Stand with your feet together, keeping your knees soft. Raise your arms alternately swinging them over your head as if you were performing backstroke.
- Raise your left arm above your head and push up as high as you can. Feel the stretch down the left side of the body. Hold for 30 seconds. Repeat on right.
- Raise your right arm to the side, keeping at shoulder height. Point your fingers towards the ceiling and push your palm away from your body. Hold for 30 seconds and repeat on left side.
- With your right hand by your side, point your fingers behind you with your palm facing up. Push your right shoulder and wrist towards the floor, then make a fist. Hold. Repeat on the other side.
- Keep your arms by your side and clench your fists as tight as you can, then spread your thumb and fingers as far apart as possible.
- Let your arms hang loosely by your side and shake them for about 15 seconds.

Back

- Clasp elbows in front of your body at shoulder height, making big circles in front of you – push out and look down. This will stretch your upper back.

- Lie on your back and raise your legs with knees bent and hands palms down at right angles to your body. Move your legs over to one side of your body keeping your knees together and bent. Repeat for the other side.
- Lie on your back with arms at right angles to your body. Raise a leg with your knee bent and let it drop over to the opposite side of your body.
- Sit back with your buttocks on your heels and head on the floor, hands outstretched in front of you. This will stretch the entire length of the spine.
- Kneel on all fours, look down whilst arching your back upwards, then slowly drop your back down and stretch your head up.
- Lie on your back with your right knee up keeping your foot on the ground. Place your left ankle on your right knee, letting your left knee drop outwards. Clasp your hands below your right knee and pull towards your body. Repeat for the other side. This will stretch the gluteals.
- Lie on your stomach with your arms by your side and gently raise your head slightly. If this feels comfortable then you can also raise your feet off the ground and raise your arms above your head in front of you. This is especially useful for straight backs and good for strengthening.

Do-In

A Self-Massage Routine To Stimulate All The Major Meridians

This is a great routine for us as massage practitioners before we start work, but it is also a suitable one to show your clients for their self-help programme. It only takes a few minutes to do, it's fun and the seriously busy people who work long hours might be willing to squeeze the sequence into their crowded daily schedule.

Stand with your feet hip-width apart and take a few deep breaths. Make a loose fist with your right hand and starting on the left shoulder, rhythmically 'punch' the muscles around the body as follows:

- Down the outside of the left arm to the hand.
- Turn the palm of your hand upwards and continue back up the inside of the arm to the armpit. (Ying channels so slightly more gently).

DO-IN FLOW

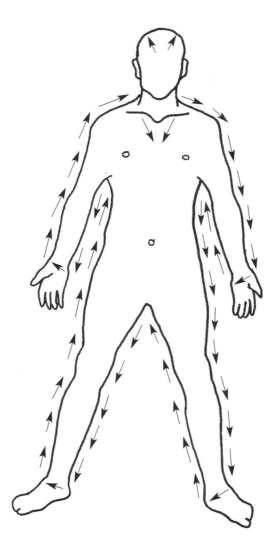

- Down the left side of body and continue down the outside of the left leg, across the top of the foot and back up the inside of the leg to the groin.
- Down the inside of the right leg over the foot and up the outside of the right leg.
- Continue up the right side of the body and down the inside of the right arm to the hand.
- Turn the right hand palm up and continue up the outside of the right arm across the top of the right shoulder.

- Beat the chest with loose fists.
- Beat the head – gently – with loose fists, starting at the top of the head at the hairline and working across the top and down to the base of the skull.
- Bend over and using the back of your fist work down either side of the spine to the gluteal muscles.
- Starting at your hands, shake your hands and arms loosely.
- Lift one leg at a time and shake loosely.
- Take three deep breaths and brush down the front and back of your body with open palms.

You will feel your energy surging round your body, you will be relaxed and clear-headed and ready to deal with your day.

A Final Word

Last but not least – A few reminders about your health and wellbeing as a practitioner:

- Pace yourself! Don't get carried away with the excitement of securing your first company contract and overextend yourself. Build in breaks for yourself between massages and try not to work on more than 12 or 13 people per day otherwise you will 'burn out'. Two or three days per week at that pace is enough for any practitioner of seated acupressure massage.
- For peace of mind, have a reliable colleague to back you up if you need a day off.
- Always eat breakfast.
- Drink plenty of filtered water.
- Consider supplementing your diet with well-balanced vitamins and minerals.
- Always stretch and ground yourself before starting treatments.
- Get a regular treatment for yourself.
- You are promoting health, so be a good rôle model for your clients and look after yourself.

The acupressure massage sequence described in detail in this book and taught in our training courses, has evolved over the years and will vary in small ways from the sequences that are taught in other accredited schools.

However, the essence of the KATA does not change. Trained practitioners in this discipline will eventually introduce elements of their own knowledge, experience and intuition to enhance their treatments, but the basic power of the KATA is always there.

It gives us enormous pleasure and satisfaction to be part of the exponential growth of interest in complementary therapies and in particular to have the opportunity to train therapists in this exciting and dynamic discipline. Many of our graduates have gone on to build successful businesses within the corporate environment and also have greatly increased their earning capacity. It is our mission to increase and develop the knowledge of seated acupressure massage amongst practitioners and to encourage them into the workplace to bring the profound benefits of the KATA to a potentially huge client base of touch-deprived, stressed-out people.

Glossary of Terms

Anma — The art of Japanese massage.

Circadian Rhythm — 24-hour biological clock.

Cosmological Sequence — Sequence of the five elements in the body.

CTD — Cumulative Trauma Disorders.

CTS — Carpal Tunnel Syndrome.

CVS — Computer Vision Syndrome.

De Quervain's Tenovaginitis — A type of Carpal Tunnel Syndrome.

Ergonomics — An applied science concerned with designing and arrangement of work environments to create maximum safety, comfort and efficiency for the worker.

Fight or Flight Mechanism — The body's release of hormones such as adrenaline and noradrenalin in response to a stressful challenge.

Five Element Theory — Taoist philosophy relating health to Growth and Control cycles of Earth, Wood, Fire, Water and Metal.

Holmes-Rahe Stress Scale — Graded scale of stressful events in life.

Huang Ti Ne Ching	Oldest existing medical text in the world.
Kata	Dance or form, used to describe the formalized moves of the 20-minute seated acupressure massage sequence. Also used in marshal arts and Tai Chi.
Ke Cycle Theory	Control Cycle of the Five Element.
Meridians	Interconnecting pathways carrying Qi (energy) to all parts of the body.
Qi or Ki (pronounced chee)	Universal life force or energy flowing through the meridians.
RSI	Repetitive Strain Injury.
Shen	Spirit.
Sheng Cycle Theory	Growth Cycle of the Five Element.
Shiatsu	'Finger pressure' massage, a derivative of Anma, now a separate discipline.
TCM	Traditional Chinese Medicine.
Tsubo	Means vase or jar in Chinese and describes the acupressure points found near the surface on the major meridians.
Types of Qi	Congenital Qi, essence of life inherited from parents at birth. Acquired Qi, derived from food we eat and air we breathe. These two combine to create Meridian Qi, Defensive Qi and Nourishing Qi. Qi in turn supports the circulation and formation of blood.

Ultradian Rhythm   The body's need for movement and a
                              change of activity every 90 minutes.

WRULD   Work-related upper limb disorders.

Yin and Yang   Opposite and balancing aspects of all of
                              life e.g. night and day, male and female,
                              cold and hot etc.

Recommended Further Reading

Health and Safety Executive: Work-related Upper Limb Disorders – A Guide to Prevention, HMSO (1990)

Holford, Patrick: Six Weeks to Super Health, Piatkus (2000) ISBN 0-7499-1963-9

Jarmey, Chris and Tindall, John: Acupressure for Common Ailments, Gaia Books (1991) ISBN 1-85675-015-9

Kushi, Michio: Natural Healing Through Macrobiotics, Japan Publications ISBN 0-87040- 457-1

Mercati, Maria: Step-by-step Tuina, Gaia Books (1997) ISBN 1-85675-038-8

Premkumar, Dr. K.: Pathology A-Z. A Handbook for Massage Therapists, Van Pub Books (2000) ISBN 0-9680730-0-X

Premkumar, Dr. K.: The Massage Connection: Anatomy, Physiology and Pathology, Van Pub Books (2000)

Pyves ,G.: No Hands Massage – Zero-Strain Bodywork, Shi'Zen Publications (2000) ISBN 0-9539074-0-6

Schneider, Meir: The Handbook of Self Healing, Penguin Books (1994) ISBN 0-14-019331-6

Bibliography and References

American Optometric Association: The Effects of Video Display Terminal Use on Eye Health and Vision, (Revised 1997)

Cash, Mel: Sports and Remedial Massage Therapy, Ebury Press (1996)

Chaitow, Leon: Muscle Energy Techniques for Muscle Dysfunction, Churchill Livingstone (1996)

Chalmers Mill, Wendy: Chartered Physiotherapist Repetitive Strain Injury, Thorsons Health Series (out of print)

Confederation of British Industry: CBI Focus on Absence Survey, CBI in conjunction with PPP (July 2000)

Gill, C.R.W.: Repetitive Strain Injury, (Update 1996)

Harvey E and Oatley, M.J.: Acupressure, Headway

Health and Safety Commission: Health and Safety Statistics, Government Statistical Service (1998)

Health and Safety Executive: Good Health is Good Business, HSE (1995)

Lewith, George T.: Acupuncture – Its Place in Western Medical Science, Thorsons (1999)

McDonald, E.: Work and Disease, (Update 1996)

Mochizuki, Shogo: Anma the Art of Japanese Massage, Kotobuki Publications (1999)

Repetitive Strain Injury Association: Newsletters, RSI Association (1998-2000)

Silk, Anne: Air Quality and the Workplace of the Future, Mid Career College Press, (1999)

Williams, Tom: Chinese Medicine, Time Life Books (1996)

Useful Addresses

The Guild of Complementary Practitioners
Liddell House, Liddell Close, Finchampstead, Berkshire RG40 4NS
Tel 0118 973 5757 Fax 0118 973 5767
e-mail info@gcpnet.com
www.gcpnet.com

RSI Association
380-384 Harrow Road, London W9 2HU
Tel: 0207 266 2000 Fax: 0207 266 2000
Helpline: 0800 018 5012

Training Schools in Seated Acupressure Massage

Seated Acupressure Massage Training School
82 The Spinney, Beaconsfield, Bucks HP9 1SA
Tel: 01494 678221 Fax: 01494 681284
e-mail abercromby@btinternet.com
www.acupressure-training.co.uk

The Academy of On-site Massage
Avon Road,Charfield,Wotton-under-Edge, Gloucestershire GL12 8TT
Tel/Fax: 01454 261900
e-mail all@onsitemassage.softnet.co.uk
www.aosm.co.uk

Touch-Pro UK
176 Melrose Avenue, London NW2 4JY
Tel: 0208 450 3366 Fax: 0208 450 2026
www.touchpro.org

Dureen Block (California USA)
www.therapure.com

European Institute of Massage
62 Greenore St, Belfast BT6 8NF, Northern Ireland
Tel: 02890 590594
e-mail jearls@eim.dndt.co.uk

There are several models of acupressure massage chairs available. Approach a training school first as most will offer a student discount.

For a list of companies/agencies offering employment to practitioners of seated acupressure massage, please contact the **Seated Acupressure Massage Training School** for details.

Appendix

Client Record Card
(These details will remain Private and Confidential)

CONSULTATION DATE: _____   CLIENT REF: _____

_____

Personal Details

NAME _____   DATE OF BIRTH _____

ADDRESS _____

_____

TEL. NO. (H) _____   TEL. NO. (W) _____

Doctor's Details

NAME _____   TEL. NO. _____

ADDRESS _____

Medical History

EPILEPSY	YES/NO	INJURIES	_____
HEART DISEASE /BP	YES/NO		_____
PREGNANT	YES/NO		_____
RECENT OPERATION	YES/NO	DETAILS	_____
RECENT FRACTURE	YES/NO	DETAILS	_____
DIGESTIVE	YES/NO	DETAILS	_____
RESPIRATORY	YES/NO	DETAILS	_____
GENITO/URINARY	YES/NO	DETAILS	_____
CIRCULATORY	YES/NO	DETAILS	_____
ALLERGIES	YES/NO	DETAILS	_____

ANY OTHER INFORMATION _____

_____

_____

General

OCCUPATION

_____

_____

STRESS LEVELS

_____

_____

GENERAL HEALTH

_____

_____

FITNESS LEVELS

_____

_____

REASON FOR MASSAGE

_____

_____

_____

_____

_____

_____

_____

Client Declaration

I am aware that this treatment is not a substitute for medical advice

I agree that to the best of my knowledge the details contained in this document are correct.

Date: _____   Signature of Client: _____

Treatment Record
(These details will remain Private and Confidential)

CLIENT REF:

Treatment Date: _____

_____

Reactions to Previous Treatment: _____

_____

_____

Aims for this Treatment: _____

_____

_____

Response to Treatment: _____

        Emotional _____

        Physical _____

Additional Notes: _____

_____

_____

_____

_____

Treatment Date: _____

_____

Reactions to Previous Treatment: _____

_____

_____

Aims for this Treatment: _____

_____

_____

Response to Treatment: _____

        Emotional _____

        Physical _____

Additional Notes: _____

_____

_____

_____

Treatment Record

(These details will remain Private and Confidential)

CLIENT REF:

_____

Treatment Date: _____

_____

Reactions to Previous Treatment: _____

_____

Aims for this Treatment: _____

_____

Response to Treatment: _____

           Emotional _____

           Physical   _____

Additional Notes: _____

_____

_____

_____

_____

Client Comments: _____

_____

_____

_____

_____

_____

_____

_____

_____

_____

_____

Signature: _____ Date: _____

Index

Notes

About The School

The Seated Acupressure Massage Training School is accredited by the Guild of Complementary Practitioners. Graduates of the School receive a Certificate of Competence that is accepted by the Guild and other professional organizations for insurance cover. Weekend and weekday courses are run year-round and throughout the UK.

For details about the training courses, dates, venues and the training video or to buy a massage chair, contact the school by phone 01494 678221, fax 01494 681284, e-mail abercromby@btinternet.com or visit the website www.acupressure-training.co.uk or write to the School at 82. The Spinney, Beaconsfield, Bucks, HP9 1SA.